Criminal Justice and Public Health

The criminal justice system now serves as the chief provider of health care services to a significant portion of society. This includes the provision of physical and mental health care for offender populations who require substantial health care resources. To date, little is known or understood with regard to how these services and programs are being delivered.

This book addresses the gaps in our knowledge by presenting a range of studies detailing the daily practices that occur in places where criminal justice and public health systems intersect. This includes an assessment of sheriff agency emergency communication systems, a study of problem behaviours and health using a juvenile sample, the challenge of treating mentally ill prison inmates with note of important gender differences, the impact of case management on justice systems, and a review of substance abuse cessation programs among pregnant women currently serving probation and parole sentences. Also included is a policy piece in which the authors call for an integrated model that is neither criminological nor public health specific. These readings provide a range of empirical examples that highlight important successes and challenges facing the criminal justice and public health systems. They suggest that integration and partnerships represent the most efficacious means to reduce critical social problems such as violence, poor health, and criminality.

This book was originally published as a special issue of *Criminal Justice Studies: A Critical Journal of Crime, Law and Society*.

Hayden Smith is an Associate Professor of Criminology and Criminal Justice at the University of South Carolina, Columbia, SC, USA. His principal research focus is the intersection of the criminal justice and public health systems. This includes self-injurious behaviour by inmates, the mental health needs of correctional populations, jail diversion, national standards of care, and premature morbidity and mortality associated with re-entry.

Criminal Justice and Public Health

Edited by

Hayden Smith

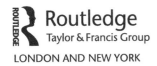

Routledge
Taylor & Francis Group

LONDON AND NEW YORK

First published 2016 by Routledge

2 Park Square, Milton Park, Abingdon, Oxon OX14 4RN
711 Third Avenue, New York, NY 10017, USA

Routledge is an imprint of the Taylor & Francis Group, an informa business

First issued in paperback 2017

Copyright © 2016 Taylor & Francis

All rights reserved. No part of this book may be reprinted or reproduced or utilised in any form or by any electronic, mechanical, or other means, now known or hereafter invented, including photocopying and recording, or in any information storage or retrieval system, without permission in writing from the publishers.

Notice:
Product or corporate names may be trademarks or registered trademarks, and are used only for identification and explanation without intent to infringe.

British Library Cataloguing in Publication Data
A catalogue record for this book is available from the British Library

ISBN 13: 978-1-138-92825-1 (hbk)
ISBN 13: 978-1-138-08646-3 (pbk)

Typeset in Times
by RefineCatch Limited, Bungay, Suffolk

Publisher's Note
The publisher accepts responsibility for any inconsistencies that may have arisen during the conversion of this book from journal articles to book chapters, namely the possible inclusion of journal terminology.

Disclaimer
Every effort has been made to contact copyright holders for their permission to reprint material in this book. The publishers would be grateful to hear from any copyright holder who is not here acknowledged and will undertake to rectify any errors or omissions in future editions of this book.

Contents

Citation Information

The following chapters were originally published in *Criminal Justice Studies: A Critical Journal of Crime, Law and Society*, volume 27, issue 1 (March 2014). When citing this material, please use the original page numbering for each article, as follows:

Editorial
Public Health & Criminal Justice
Hayden Smith
Criminal Justice Studies: A Critical Journal of Crime, Law and Society, volume 27, issue 1 (March 2014) pp. 1–3

Chapter 1
Assessing sheriff's office emergency and disaster website communications
Philip Matthew Stinson Sr., John Liederbach, L. Fleming Fallon Jr. and Hans Schmalzried
Criminal Justice Studies: A Critical Journal of Crime, Law and Society, volume 27, issue 1 (March 2014) pp. 4–19

Chapter 2
Exploring gender differences in constellations of problem behaviors and associated health-related factors during adolescence
Kristina K. Childs
Criminal Justice Studies: A Critical Journal of Crime, Law and Society, volume 27, issue 1 (March 2014) pp. 20–42

Chapter 3
The effects of treatment exposure on prison misconduct for female prisoners with substance use, mental health, and co-occurring disorders
Kimberly A. Houser, Brandy L. Blasko and Steven Belenko
Criminal Justice Studies: A Critical Journal of Crime, Law and Society, volume 27, issue 1 (March 2014) pp. 43–62

Chapter 4
Correctional outcomes of offenders with mental disorders
Lynn A. Stewart and Geoff Wilton
Criminal Justice Studies: A Critical Journal of Crime, Law and Society, volume 27, issue 1 (March 2014) pp. 63–81

Chapter 5

Service utilization in a cohort of criminal justice-involved men: implications for case management and justice systems
Roberto Hugh Potter
Criminal Justice Studies: A Critical Journal of Crime, Law and Society, volume 27, issue 1 (March 2014) pp. 82–95

Chapter 6

Influences on substance use cessation during pregnancy: an exploratory study of women on probation and parole
Rebecca J. Stone and Merry Morash
Criminal Justice Studies: A Critical Journal of Crime, Law and Society, volume 27, issue 1 (March 2014) pp. 96–113

Chapter 7

Moving prison health promotion along: towards an integrative framework for action to develop health promotion and tackle the social determinants of health
James Woodall, Nick de Viggiani, Rachael Dixey and Jane South
Criminal Justice Studies: A Critical Journal of Crime, Law and Society, volume 27, issue 1 (March 2014) pp. 114–132

Please direct any queries you may have about the citations to
clsuk.permissions@cengage.com

Notes on Contributors

Steven Belenko is Professor in the Department of Criminal Justice at Temple University, Philadelphia, PA, USA. His research interests focus on the implementation of evidence-based treatment and other services into the criminal justice and juvenile justice systems, the impact of substance abuse and other health problems on the adult and juvenile justice systems, and developing and testing organizational change strategies to improve implementation of treatment and other health services for offenders. He has also authored and edited several books.

Brandy L. Blasko is a Postdoctoral Research Fellow at George Mason University, Fairfax, Virginia, USA, with a joint appointment in the Department of Criminology, Law and Society and the Department of Psychology. Her research focuses on discretion and decision making, prison policymaking, and offender rehabilitation.

Kristina K. Childs is an Assistant Professor in the Department of Criminal Justice at the University of Central Florida, Orlando, FL, USA. Her primary research interests include juvenile justice system policy, prevention and intervention strategies for juvenile offenders, and understanding the intersection of public health and juvenile justice-related services.

Nick de Viggiani is a Senior Lecturer at the University of the West of England, Bristol, UK. His PhD research (1999–2003) entailed an ethnographic study of masculinities and health within an English prison. He led the South West Offender Health Research Network in England for five years and has led several funded research projects within justice settings, the most recent a project in partnership with a national music charity involving young people in justice contexts. He has a keen interest in advancing and reorienting public health within justice systems, and he has a strong publication record in the field of justice health.

Rachael Dixey is a Professor of Health Promotion at Leeds Beckett University, UK. She recently finished writing and editing a book on health promotion, conceptualising it as a broad social movement aimed at social justice in health and tackling the inequalities and inequities in health. Her other recent research includes examining the concept of healthy prisons, and issues facing the families of prisoners, subjects on which she has several recent publications.

L. Fleming Fallon Jr. is Distinguished Teaching Professor and Director of Public Health in the Department of Public and Allied Health at Bowling Green State University, Ohio, USA. He is the author of ten books and more than 80 articles in scholarly journals.

Kimberly A. Houser is a Professor in the Department of Criminal Justice at Kutztown University, PA, USA. She is also an Adjunct Professor in the Criminal Justice Department at Temple University, Philadelphia, PA, USA. Her research interests include co-occurring and mental health disorders in the offender population, re-entry and reintegration of offenders, and substance abuse treatment.

John Liederbach is an Associate Professor in the Criminal Justice Program at Bowling Green State University, Ohio, USA. His primary research interests include the study of police behaviour across community types, suburban and rural policing, police corruption and crime, and white collar crime.

Merry Morash is Professor in the School of Criminal Justice, Michigan State University, East Lansing, MI, USA. Her recent books include *Women on Probation and Parole: A Feminist Critique of Community Programs and Services*, and *Understanding Gender, Crime and Justice*. Along with Meda Chesney Lind, she also is editor of the edited volume, *Feminist Theories of Crime*. In addition to domestic violence among immigrant populations, her current research focuses on an integrated theory of communication and corrections applied to women on probation, girls in juvenile court, and the influence of school context on delinquency.

Roberto Hugh Potter is a Sociologist and Criminologist currently working at the intersection of criminal justice, public health and the community. His current work focuses on the operations of the criminal justice and community systems, from primary to tertiary prevention of criminal behaviour, injury, and infectious diseases. He has worked as a State and Federal researcher and manager; as a manager in the community-based organisational sector; and as an academic at US and Australian universities.

Hans Schmalzried is a Professor of Public Health and serves as Chair of the Department of Public and Allied Health at Bowling Green State University, Ohio, USA. He previously served concurrently (1987–2005) as Health Officer for two county health districts (Fulton County, Ohio and Henry County, Ohio). Prior to this, he spent seven years (1980–1987) as an Environmental Scientist and Engineer with the Ohio Environmental Protection Agency.

Hayden Smith is an Associate Professor of Criminology and Criminal Justice at the University of South Carolina, Columbia, SC, USA. His principal research focus is the intersection of the criminal justice and public health systems. This includes self-injurious behaviour by inmates, the mental health needs of correctional populations, jail diversion, national standards of care, and premature morbidity and mortality associated with re-entry.

Jane South is a Professor of Healthy Communities at Leeds Beckett University, UK. She has a national and international reputation for her research on lay health workers and volunteer roles in health. She has a long standing interest in community engagement and is the lead author of the recently published 'People-Centred Public Health'. She recently led an NIHR funded research study examining the effectiveness and cost-effectiveness of peer interventions in prison.

Lynn A. Stewart is a Senior Research Manager at the Correctional Service of Canada. She has authored government reports and journal articles related to correctional program outcomes, offenders with mental health and chronic health disorders, and domestic violence perpetration and treatment. She has co-authored treatment program curricula for violent women and general offending programs for male offenders.

Philip Matthew Stinson Sr. is an Assistant Professor in the Criminal Justice Program at Bowling Green State University, Ohio, USA. His primary research interests include the study of police crime and police integrity, and he is currently principal investigator in a national study of police integrity funded by the National Institute of Justice at the US Department of Justice.

Rebecca J. Stone is a Doctoral Candidate in the School of Criminal Justice at Michigan State University, East Lansing, MI, USA. She also holds a Master of Public Health degree from Michigan State University. Her research focuses on the nexus of public health and criminal justice, especially issues concerning women, substance use, and access to health care. Her other topics of interest include violence against women, health care for criminal justice populations, and qualitative studies of desistance from offending.

Geoff Wilton joined the Correctional Service of Canada as a Researcher in 2009 after completing his studies at Carleton University, Ottawa, Canada. His primary research interests are in the areas of the effectiveness of correctional interventions and on outcomes of offenders with mental health problems. He has co-authored articles in peer review journals and numerous government research reports.

James Woodall is a Senior Lecturer and the co-Director of the Centre for Health Promotion Research at Leeds Beckett University, UK. His PhD explored the health promoting prison and how values central to health promotion are applied to the context of imprisonment. He has published on a number of subjects, including prisoners' lay views on health, the mental health of prisoners and young offenders, the role of prison visitors' centres in reducing health inequalities and the health needs of prison staff.

Dedication

This book is dedicated to Neil Patrick Smith and Patricia Ella Smith.
There are three things that parents deserve to hear.

I love you both deeply
I am proud to call you my Dad and Mum
You were right all along…

INTRODUCTION
Public Health & Criminal Justice

The following special edition of *Criminal Justice Studies* centers on issues that intersect both the criminal justice and public health systems. It relies on a longstanding World Health Organization's definition of public health as, 'a state of complete physical, mental and social well-being and not merely the absence of disease or infirmity' (1948). Using this approach, health is categorized into a tripartite schema that involves the nexus of the physical body, the mind, and consideration of broader society. These components are particularly salient for the modern day criminal justice system where front-line workers are legally responsible for providing health, safety, and access to treatment to both offenders and their victims on a daily basis.

In terms of physical health, individuals who regularly interact with the criminal justice system disproportionately share the burden of infectious disease and poor health; with the presence of an extensive criminal history remaining a strong predictor of physical illness. With regard to mental health, the failures of the deinstitutionalization movement have produced a vulnerable social group who receive their housing, food, psychiatric assessment, medication, and therapy entirely within the criminal justice system. In the United States context, this has resulted in the three largest mental health institutions now being correctional facilities. The offenders housed within these institutions (i.e. New York's Riker's Island, Chicago's Cook County Jail and the Los Angeles County Jail) and others disproportionately exhibit high rates of psychiatric morbidity when compared to their non-incarcerated counterparts. Such disparities are more observable within the prison context, with inmates commonly experiencing symptoms associated with severe and persistent mental illnesses that are difficult to manage. The final component of social health centers on the relationship between ecological variables and poor community health. While frequent and serious crime is certainly an indicator of a dysfunctional neighborhood, criminality occurs within a real world setting that is often rife with additional impediments to health. This includes recognition of distal issues such as economic inequality, racism, gangs, political pandering, white collar crime, globalization, and a lack of access to quality education, nutrition, and basic health care.

The responsibility of providing physical, mental, and social health resources for a segment of society have now been largely adopted, or rather forced upon the criminal justice system. Although it is neither surprising nor accidental that criminal justice and public health systems have become increasingly enmeshed. In 1985, surgeon General C. Everett Koop convened his Workshop on Violence and Public Health conference which signaled public health's first foray into violence prevention. This meeting featured 11 working groups that explored issues that were historically restricted to the domain of criminal justice. Examples include homicide, spousal abuse, and sexual assault. Koop made it clear that the mission of public health would continue to expand in order to address other social pathologies. Since that time, there has been a growing recognition that criminal justice and public health systems continue to address very similar populations who have very similar problems; and that these problems are becomingly increasingly complex and expensive to treat. While organic or 'grass root' partnerships occur between criminal justice and public health staff on an ad hoc basis; there is also a need to address these issues empirically, thus the need for this special edition. The following studies have been conducted by a range of criminologists and public health experts within the international community. This participation of various academicians suggests that the research in this special edition is actually driving at a global phenomenon, one in which synchronicity of these differing systems is inevitable. I will now briefly discuss some of the highlights within these articles.

In the first article, Stinson and colleagues present a content analysis of sheriff's office website homepages using a nine-point scale to measure emergency communication. They identify the presence or absence of important communication elements on these websites' and provide policy suggestions. This study offers insight into the need for effective communication in supporting readiness for public health emergencies. While terrorist events and natural disasters are inevitable, this study reveals that much more work is needed in order for sheriff agencies to deliver information regarding such events.

The second article by Kristina Childs explores the intersection of juvenile justice and public health services. This features an examination of the relationship between problem behavior and general health in a sample of juvenile delinquents. Childs identifies key latent constructs and notes important gender differences. This study is particularly relevant for systems in which juveniles exhibit behavioral issues and health deficits that can overwhelm institutional resources.

The next two articles by Houser, Blasko, & Belenko and Stewart & Wilton examine mental health in the prison context. Houser, Blasko, and Belenko assessed a sample of female offenders with co-occurring disorders of mental health and substance abuse. They highlight the impact of mental illness on treatment length and misconduct sanctions. Stewart and Wilton provide a portrait of mentally ill offenders in Canada. They draw attention to the higher risk and needs rating of these offenders, particularly the higher rates of institutional charges and transfers to segregation for offenders with a mental disorder. Both studies suggest that inmates who have a mental illness experience prison quite differently from other inmates who do not have a mental illness.

In article five, Hugh Potter studies the intersection of case management and justice systems. Specifically, Potter looked at pre-incarceration utilization of services and finds that HIV testing is one area in which services are used efficiently. Policy implications are provided for other services which seem to be lacking. This is followed by a study of probation and parole systems by Rebecca Stone and Merry Morash. Stone and Morash examine substance abuse cessation among a sample of pregnant women who were on probation or parole. The concept of self-efficacy is emphasized in their policy recommendations.

The final article by Woodall and his colleagues is a policy-assessment piece that argues that neither a strict criminological nor public health model will be sufficient for change. The authors call for an integrated model and cite the Ottawa Charter as an exemplar of success. The often undervalued goal of social health is explained as being possible through partnerships that feature diverse academic and practitioner orientations.

Combined, these articles feature a wealth of thought-provoking approaches, innovative methods, and germane policy implications. Note that I have only provided a cursory description of these articles in order to encourage the reader to access each study themself. Of course, like all good research, these studies raise more questions for the future. For example, one common theme discussed in all of these studies involves the blurring of traditional roles for criminal justice staff. Consider the following collection of such questions from this special edition; 'Should sheriffs define themselves as "crime fighters" or "emergency responders"?'; 'If subsets of adolescent boys and girls display high levels of problem behaviors and health deficiencies, can juvenile justice staff effectively treat them?'; 'Do correctional staff require "cross-training" in order to address the complex needs of mentally ill and substance dependent inmates?'; 'How should correctional staff treat inmates who have a serious mental illness, which also includes acts of violence'; 'How can staff best provide pre- and post-incarceration health services when confronted with social issues like homelessness?'; 'How can probation and parole officers promote drug use resistance in pregnant women, who may also have mental health problems and a lack of family support?' These are challenging questions that certainly warrant more research.

The articles in this special edition highlight criminal justice systems that continue to serve as a proxy public health care system for many of our citizens. This is particularly daunting when one considers that the criminal justice system was created for the singular purpose of protecting the public order. However, academicians can ease this integration of the criminal justice and public health systems by conducting empirical research on what works and what does not work. We have already seen progressive and documented change in public health-related policies; with police receiving Memphis model training for dealing with the mentally ill, court systems now featuring specialized drug addiction and mental health courts, and corrections increasing education, training, and intervention programming. These changes can only be bolstered by the articles in this special edition, which hopefully provide the reader with a portrait of how public health issues are currently being addressed within the criminal justice system. I hope you enjoy reading them as much as I did.

As a final note, I would like to extend a sincere appreciation to the anonymous reviewers of these studies. These reviewer experts came from both criminal justice and public health fields of study and devoted their time to improving the quality of these articles. I would also like to thank the Editor of *Criminal Justice Studies*, Dr Richard Tewksbury, for making this special edition possible.

Reference

World Health Organization. (1948). Definition of health. *Preamble to the Constitution of the World Health Organization as adopted by the International Health Conference*, New York, NY, June 19–22, 1946; signed on July 22, 1946 by the representatives of 61 States (official records of the World Health Organization, no. 2, p. 100) and entered into force on April 7, 1948.

Hayden Smith

Assessing sheriff's office emergency and disaster website communications

Philip Matthew Stinson Sr., John Liederbach, L. Fleming Fallon Jr. and
Hans Schmalzried

Criminal Justice Program, Bowling Green State University, Bowling Green, OH, USA

Sheriff's offices are an integral component of the public health emergency preparedness and response system in the USA. During a public health emergency or disaster, sheriff's offices need to communicate with people affected by the event. Sheriff's office websites are logical sources for information about disaster preparedness and response efforts. No prior research evaluates emergency preparedness and response resources available through sheriff's office websites. The current research is a national study of sheriff's office websites to assess the availability of information relating to emergency preparedness and response. A content analysis of 2590 sheriff's office website homepages was conducted to determine the presence or absence of nine communications elements important to people seeking information during an emergency or disaster. We found that 71.9% of sheriff's office website homepages include links to agency services and programs, but only 6.5% provide links to emergency preparedness information. The findings of the study are useful to assess emergency preparedness and the amount of response information available, as well as to identify opportunities to improve sheriff's office website homepages.

Responses to emergencies and disasters require the dissemination of specific and reliable information to the public, including communication on what to do, where to go, and what help is available. The Internet has increasingly become the prime vehicle to inform individuals and society, as well as victims, about preparing and coping during and after emergencies and disasters (Hobbs, Kittler, Fox, Middleton, & Bates, 2004). In the USA, more than three out of four households (76.7%) have a computer with access to the Internet (US Census Bureau, 2012). Nearly half of all American adults (46%) own a smartphone that provides Internet connectivity and web browsing capability (Smith, 2012). Although traditional media outlets remain an important source of information, the Internet provides news and content that is more easily and quickly accessible for many citizens – so much so that websites and their content can directly affect the overall quality of emergency responses and determine how well victims and the public are served during and in the aftermath of emergencies and disasters.

Emergency communications in the form of web-based content involve a network of public and private entities that includes the office of the sheriff. The sheriff has been identified as a key player within the domains of public health emergency response (McCabe, Barnett, Taylor, & Links, 2010; McKing, 2008), emergency preparedness (Drake, 2009; Giblin, Schafer, & Burruss, 2009; Wholey, Gregg, & Moscovice, 2009), homeland security (Oliver, 2009; Pelfrey, 2009), dissemination of information to increase citizen preparedness (Burch, 2012), and the prevention of terrorism (Pelfrey, 2007). Dating from 900 years of tradition that traces its roots to medieval England, sheriff's offices in the USA employ over 353,000 personnel, including 182,000 sworn officers (Reaves, 2011). The importance of this popularly elected office within the American policing institution and the realm of emergency preparedness stems from the sheriff's unique historical and organizational character, particularly the office's broad scope of legal authority and county-level jurisdiction (Falcone & Wells, 1995; Liederbach & Frank, 2006). The sheriff has evolved into a 'multi-purpose office' with a broader range of responsibilities than those performed by municipal police agencies (Falcone & Wells, 1995, p. 130). The sheriff's prime responsibility is that of *conservator of the peace* as the chief law enforcement officer in the county. This function includes the role of public safety director and the promotion of public safety at the county level (Struckhoff & Scott, 2003). Most sheriff's offices are responsible for serving civil process and providing court security, and in many states the county sheriff's office operates the county jail and/or provides general law enforcement patrols of the unincorporated areas (Hickman & Reaves, 2006). Half of all sheriff's offices employ full-time school resource officers (Burch, 2012). The public can reach most sheriffs' offices by dialing enhanced 9-1-1 systems capable of displaying a caller's name, location, and special needs (Burch, 2012).

During an emergency or disaster, sheriff's offices need to communicate with citizens affected by the event, and sheriff's websites are logical sources for information about disaster preparedness and response efforts. We are aware of no published research, however, that evaluate emergency preparedness resources available through sheriff's websites. These data are integral to an overall assessment of the content and quality of information available to the public during emergencies and disasters given the sheriff's role as the county-level public safety director and the fact that websites have become an important informational resource during these scenarios. The current research is a national study of sheriff's websites and information relative to emergency preparedness. We analyzed the content of website homepages for 2590 sheriff's offices for the presence or absence of nine communication elements important to citizens seeking information during and in the immediate aftermath of a disaster or emergency. These data can be used to assess informational communications available to citizens on sheriff's websites as well as identify opportunities to improve these websites and the provision of information and emergency services to the public.

Literature review

No published studies assessing sheriff's websites for effectiveness of communications during an emergency or disaster could be found in the literature; however, there are two areas that provide a relevant context for the current study including: (a) literature on the role and function of the sheriff during emergencies and disasters, and (b) research on the identification of key elements of effective websites, particularly those studies focused on the evaluation of emergency preparedness resources available on the Internet.

The sheriff and emergency response

The sheriff has been largely overlooked as a subject of study by scholars (Helms, 2008; LaFrance & Placide, 2010). Policing scholars have ignored sheriffs and instead portrayed the large urban municipal police department as the dominant mode of policing in the USA (Falcone & Wells, 1995; Liederbach & Frank, 2006). This gap in the literature is no small consideration given the vast organizational and functional differences between these offices and the more-often studied urban municipal agency. First, the sheriff derives authority directly through public election rather than administrative appointment. The political nature of the position supports open communication between the office and the public, as well as coordination between the sheriff and other social service agencies (Falcone & Wells, 1995). Second, sheriffs and their deputy officers typically patrol within a much larger geographic area than municipal police officers, including unincorporated rural areas and/or those having overlapping jurisdiction within local municipalities. Third, the sheriff has historically been entrusted with a broader range of responsibilities than those performed by municipal agencies. Similar to the historical *shire-reeve*, the modern office of sheriff typically performs several functions in addition to traditional law enforcement, including court services, civil process and writs, correctional administration, and the collection of taxes and fees (Brown, 1989). Struckhoff and Scott (2003) emphasize the degree of variation across these offices nationwide, and the fact that sheriff's operating in smaller nonmetropolitan or rural counties differ from those who 'report to an office in a skyscraper and manage an office whose budget exceeds that of many corporations or cities' (p. 68).

Despite these variations, the office of sheriff typically operates as a county-wide law enforcement agency that holds the potential for coordinating efforts designed to mitigate and respond to emergencies and disasters, such as the maintenance of county and civil law enforcement operations, search and rescue, perimeter security, and victim assistance (Hickman & Reaves, 2006). These traditional roles have expanded in the aftermath of the 2001 terrorist attacks and federal strategies designed to improve emergency preparedness and mitigate threats posed by terrorism (Murray, 2005; Pelfrey, 2007). Many agencies have recently developed sheriff's emergency response teams to deal with emergencies that occur both inside and outside the jail system, including those that involve hazardous materials and natural disasters (Strandberg, 2004). Likewise, the National Sheriff's Association's (NSA) Institute for Homeland Security provides training in homeland protection to emergency responders including sheriff's deputies to become Certified Homeland Protection Professionals who specialize in the prevention and mitigation of all types of emergencies and disasters (NSA, 2012).

Evaluation of emergency preparedness resources on the Internet

Studies on websites operated within the retail industry provide a basis for understanding how website design and content influences the user experience. For example, website content that is current and maintained by experts appears to contribute to success (Yen, 2007); but, poor website design can frustrate users and cause them to leave without making a purchase (Tan & Wei, 2006; Yeung & Lu, 2004). Although many features of retail websites are not immediately applicable to sheriff's websites, there is an emerging line of research focused on the evaluation of emergency preparedness resources on the Internet. These studies can be used to identify key elements critical for effective communications during emergencies and disasters and points of comparison between websites operated by sheriffs and those operated by other types of agencies, including local health departments (LHD) (Fallon, Schmalzried, & Hasan, 2011), local emergency management agencies (EMA) (Schmalzried, Fallon, Keller, & McHugh, 2011), and local chapters of the American Red Cross (ARC) (Schmalzried, Fleming Fallon, & Harper, 2012).

These studies identified key elements for effective online communications during emergencies and disasters that were adapted from the criteria used by Kim, Eng, Deering, and Maxfield (1999) to assess health-related websites. Fallon, Schmalzried, and Hasan (2011) analyzed the content of websites operated by LHD based on the presence or absence of nine elements deemed to be critical for effective communications during emergencies or disasters. They found that four of five (80.5%) of LHD website homepages included the agency phone number, half (49.4%) provided links to emergency information, and one in five (19.6%) listed an agency email address. Less than one in 20 (4.3%) of the LHD homepages allowed visitors to sign up for automatic alerts or notifications. Schmalzried et al. (2011) analyzed websites operated by local EMA and found that the content of these websites were similar to those operated by LHDs in terms of the inclusion of agency phone number (82.3%) and links to emergency information (52%). Homepages operated by EMAs, however, were much more likely to list an agency email address (38.3%) and/or allow users to sign up for alerts or notifications (21.1%). Schmalzried et al. (2012) analyzed websites operated by local chapters of the ARC. ARC homepages were more likely to include an organizational logo (95.7%) and/or allow users to sign up for alerts or notifications (23%) than either LHDs or EMAs. ARC homepages provided links to other disaster relief/emergency preparedness organizations or information (32%) less commonly than LHDs (49.4%) or EMAs (52%).

Method

A nationwide list of 3,063 sheriff offices was obtained from the Census of State and Local Law Enforcement Agencies (CSLLEA) (US Department of Justice, 2008). We utilized the nine-point scale developed by Fallon, Schmalzried, and Hasan to indicate the presence or absence of important communication elements on these websites (Fallon et al., 2011; Schmalzried et al., 2011, 2012). Table 1 presents an overview of the evolution of essential communication elements derived in part from the guiding principles of emergency communications, and the corresponding webpage criteria developed by Kim et al. (1999). The right-most column in Table 1 lists the nine sheriff-specific website communication elements used in the current study. The homepage for each of the identified sheriff's offices were examined to determine the presence or absence of these elements: (1) organization logo (star-shaped sheriff badge), (2) date the website was last modified, (3) name of the top agency executive, (4) links to agency programs/services, (5) links to emergency preparedness information, (6) state where agency is located, (7) agency

Table 1. Evolution of essential communication elements.

Guiding principles	Webpage criteria developed by Kim et al.	Corresponding elements
Establishing credibility	Disclosure of authors, sponsors, developers (includes identification of purpose, nature of organization, sources of support, authorship, origin)	Organization logo (star-shaped sheriff badge)
Providing frequent and up-to-date information	Currency of information (including frequency of update, freshness, maintenance of site)	Date the web-site was last modified
Demonstrating leadership	Authority of source (includes reputation of source, credibility, trustworthiness)	Name of top agency executive
Collaborating with other organizations	Links (includes quality of links, links to other sources)	Links to agency programs/ services & links to emergency preparedness info
Defining who is being served	Intended audience (includes nature of intended users, appropriateness for intended users)	State where agency is located
Ensuring multiple channels of information	Contact addresses or feedback mechanism (includes availability of contact information, contact address)	Agency phone number and email
Providing reassurance	User support (includes availability of support and documentation of users)	Availability to sign up for automatic alert/notification

phone number, (8) agency email, and (9) availability to sign up for automatic alert/ notification.

Analytic strategy

A quantitative content analysis was conducted of sheriff's website homepages to determine the presence or absence of nine communication elements important to citizens seeking information during and in the immediate aftermath of a disaster or emergency. Content analysis is a research methodology for making valid and reli-able inferences from textual or other meaningful content to the contexts of their use (Krippendorff, 2013). Content analysis research involves a process where trained coders record their observation counts of specific units or variables on coding instruments based on predetermined coding definitions. Through this coding process each coder is inferring features of a nonmanifest context – in this case, emergency communication elements – from features of a manifest text. Content analysis is appropriate for this study because it provides a rigorous methodological framework allowing for replication using the nine-point scale developed by Fallon, Schmalzried, and Hasan (2011), Schmalzried et al. (2011, 2012) to extend their research on website communications in public health emergencies in the context of sheriff's office website homepages.

Coding was completed over a three-month period beginning in March 2012 and involved two individual coders who were trained by one of the authors on the coding protocol and use of the coding instrument. Each of the coders was provided a list of one-half of the sheriff offices on the CSLLEA list. The coders utilized the Google® search engine to locate the official website homepage of the sheriff agencies. Coders indicated the presence or absence of each of the essential communication elements on the website homepages. Coders also indicated whether the homepages included links to a sheriff office's Facebook® page and/or Twitter® address. We also recorded information on the state (using the 50 states and the District of Columbia), a measure of rurality using the US Department of Agriculture's nine-point Rural-Urban Continuum Codes (US Department of Agriculture, 2003), as well as a variable from the CSLEEA that captured the number of full-time sworn employees in the sheriff offices and another that differentiated between those agencies providing routine patrol services and those agencies that do not provide routine patrol services. Coded data were recorded in an SPSS® data set for analysis. Completed coding instruments were scanned into encrypted digital PDF files for safekeeping.

Analytic procedures were undertaken to ensure reliability of the data. A third coder was employed to independently code a random sample of 5% of the total number of cases. The overall level of simple agreement between the three coders across the variables of interest in this study (88.45%) established a degree of reliability generally considered acceptable (see Riffe, Lacy, & Fico, 2005). Reliability was also computed for the nine variables making up the communication element scale using Krippendorf's alpha (see Hayes & Krippendorff, 2007). The Krippendorf's alpha coefficient is strong across communication element variables (Krippendorf's $\alpha = .765$). The intercoder reliability coding was performed in July 2012, several months after the primary coders completed their content analysis coding of website home pages. It is possible that some websites changed during this four-month period, as web content is not static and sites are constantly being revised, content changes, and elements evolve over time. The alpha coefficient calculated may reflect such changes over time and may not be indicative of problematic coder reliability.

Strengths and limitations of the data

There are no published studies assessing the degree to which local sheriff's effectively communicate during an emergency or disaster – despite the sheriff's integral role in emergency preparedness as the chief law enforcement officer within the vast majority of counties in the USA. This study fills this important gap in the scholarly literature using a methodology that allows data collection from sheriff's offices from across the nation. The study also utilizes a multidimensional measure of emergency preparedness and response resources available through the sheriff's websites. The methodology explores a form of communication that has and continues to gain prominence within emergency response networks.

These data have two primary limitations. First, the content analysis of website homepages does not assess other factors that likely indicate the degree to which local sheriff's may or may not communicate during an emergency or disaster. It is likely, for example, that large sheriff's offices devote more resources to the production of high-quality websites than do sheriffs in rural counties where face-to-face interaction and more informal forms of communication may be more likely or even preferable to websites for the communication of emergency information. It is also possible that a website might not be available during an emergency. Second, the identification of official sheriff's websites was complicated by the existence of numerous 'shadow' or nonofficial websites promulgated by candidates for the office of sheriff that were constructed to support upcoming political campaigns. These websites were not part of the official sheriff's website and were hosted on commercial servers with nongovernmental uniform resource locators (URL). These 'shadow' websites were subsequently identified and excluded from the analyses.

Results

A homepage for the official agency website was located for 2590 (84.5%) of the 3063 sheriff's offices in 46 states that participated in the 2008 CSLLEA survey. Four states (Alaska, Connecticut, Hawaii, and Rhode Island) and the District of Columbia do not have local sheriffs. Included in the sample are 30 city sheriff's offices for independent cities.[1] The results of the content analysis of website homepages are initially presented in terms of frequencies and percentages of the homepage communication elements for the entire sample, and measures of central tendency and dispersion for the entire sample. We also present the homepage communication elements disaggregated in terms of metropolitan vs. nonmetropolitan sheriff's offices given that previous literature highlights the degree of variation across sheriff's offices nationwide and apparent differences between offices that operate in rural jurisdictions and those in urban and/or suburban areas (see Hickman & Reaves, 2006; Reaves, 2011).

Table 2 demonstrates that four communication elements appeared on most websites including: (a) state where the local law enforcement agency is located ($n = 2376$, 91.7%), (b) name of the top agency executive ($n = 2292$, 88.5%), (c) agency phone number ($n = 2166$, 83.6%), and (d) links to agency programs or services ($n = 1862$, 71.9%). Approximately one-third of the websites listed the sheriff star-shaped badge as an organizational logo ($n = 971$, 37.5%) and the email address of the agency ($n = 846$, 32.7%). The remainder of communication elements appeared much less frequently including availability to sign up for automatic alert/notification ($n = 328$, 12.7%), date the website was last modified ($n = 170$, 6.6%), and links to emergency preparedness information ($n = 168$, 6.5%).

Measures of central tendency and dispersion are presented in Table 3. The mean number of communication elements found was $\bar{X} = 4.3$ (SD = 1.17). The median number of communication elements found was 4. The maximum number of

Table 2. Sheriff agency homepage communication elements ($N = 2590$).

Rank	Agency communication elements	n	%
1	State where agency is located	2376	91.7
2	Name of top agency executive	2292	88.5
3	Agency phone number	2166	83.6
4	Links to agency programs/services	1862	71.9
5	Organization logo (star-shaped sheriff badge)	971	37.5
6	Email address of agency	846	32.7
7	Availability to sign up for automatic alert/notification	328	12.7
8	Date the website was last modified	170	6.6
9	Links to emergency preparedness information	168	6.5

Table 3. Web-site communication elements.

Measure	Value
Mean	4.32
Standard deviation	1.177
Median	4
Range	7
Minimum	1
Maximum	8

Table 4. Sheriff offices communication elements present on homepage: bivariate associations with metro vs. non-metro counties ($N = 2590$).

Agency communication elements	Metro county ($n = 987$)			Non-metro county ($n = 1603$)			χ^2	df	p	V
	n	Agency (%)	%	n	Agency (%)	%				
State where agency is located	881	(89.3)	37.1	1495	(93.3)	62.9	12.909	1	<.001	.071
Agency phone number	782	(79.2)	36.1	1384	(86.3)	63.9	22.544	1	<.001	.093
Email address of agency	282	(28.6)	33.3	564	(35.2)	66.7	12.133	1	<.001	.068
Name of top executive	882	(89.4)	38.5	1410	(87.9)	61.5	1.179	1	.278	.021
Links to agency programs/ services	839	(85.0)	45.1	1023	(63.8)	54.9	135.702	1	<.001	.229
Links to emergency preparedness information	79	(8.0)	47.0	89	(5.5)	53.0	6.055	1	.014	.048
Availability to sign up for automatic alert/ notification	137	(13.9)	41.8	191	(11.9)	58.2	2.133	1	.144	.029
Date website was last modified	61	(6.2)	35.9	109	(6.8)	64.1	0.382	1	.536	.012
Organizational logo (star-shaped sheriff badge)	494	(50.0)	50.9	477	(29.8)	49.1	107.354	1	<.001	.204

communication elements found was 8 and the minimum number of communication elements found was 1.

Table 4 shows how the content of website homepages for agencies located in metropolitan counties compared with those of agencies located in nonmetropolitan counties. We identified 986 sheriff's offices in metropolitan counties and 1601 sheriff's offices in nonmetropolitan counties. Sheriff's offices located in metropolitan counties were statistically more likely to include links to agency programs and services (85.0%) on their website homepage than were sheriff's offices located in nonmetropolitan rural counties (63.8%). Similarly, sheriff's offices located in metropolitan counties more often included on their website homepage a star-shaped sheriff's badge as an organizational logo (50%) than were sheriff agencies located in rural nonmetropolitan counties (29.8%). Sheriff's offices located in nonmetropolitan counties were more likely to include agency phone number and/or email address than agencies located in metropolitan counties. The bivariate associations for the remaining communication elements were statistically insignificant at the $p < .05$ level, meaning that sheriff's offices in nonmetropolitan counties were just as likely as sheriff's offices located in metropolitan counties to include on their website homepage the name of their top executive, the ability to sign up for automatic alerts/notifications, and the date website was last modified.

Table 5 presents the website homepage emergency communications elements for sheriff's offices providing routine patrol services compared to those sheriff's offices that do not provide routine patrol services. Sheriff's offices that provide routine patrol services were statistically more likely to include links to emergency preparedness information (6.4%) than were sheriff's offices not providing the provision of routine patrol services (2.0%). Likewise, sheriff's offices that provide routine patrol services were also more likely to provide the ability to sign up for automatic alerts and notifications (12.4%) than were sheriff's offices not providing routine patrol services (6.9%). The bivariate associations for the other seven communications elements were statistically insignificant at the $p < .05$ level, meaning that those sheriff's offices not providing routine patrol services were just as likely as those sheriff's offices providing routine patrol services to include the other elements (i.e. state where located, agency phone number, agency email address, name of top executive, star-shaped sheriff badge logo, and date website was last modified) on their website homepage.[2]

Table 5. Sheriff offices communication elements present on homepage: bivariate associations with routine patrol services ($N = 2574$).

Agency communication elements	Provides routine patrol services						χ^2	df	p	V
	Yes ($n = 2531$)			No ($n = 143$)						
	n	Agency (%)	%	n	Agency (%)	%				
State where agency is located	2230	(86.6)	94.5	130	(90.9)	5.5	0.120	1	.729	.007
Agency phone number	2038	(80.5)	94.7	113	(79.0)	5.3	2.278	1	.131	.030
Email address of agency	792	(31.3)	94.3	48	(33.5)	5.7	0.060	1	.807	.005
Name of top executive	2152	(85.0)	94.6	124	(86.7)	5.4	0.432	1	.511	.013
Links to agency programs/ services	1742	(68.8)	94.2	108	(75.5)	5.8	0.999	1	.318	.020
Links to emergency preparedness information	164	(6.4)	98.2	3	(2.0)	1.8	4.810	1	.028	.043
Availability to sign up for automatic alert/notification	315	(12.4)	96.9	10	(6.9)	3.1	4.355	1	.037	.041
Date website was last modified	162	(6.4)	95.3	8	(5.6)	4.7	0.250	1	.617	.010
Organizational logo (star-shaped sheriff badge)	909	(35.9)	94.2	56	(39.1)	5.8	0.180	1	.671	.008

Discussion

Recent events reinforce the critical importance of clear and readily available information during emergencies and disasters – from the devastated beach-front communities paralyzed in the wake of Hurricane Sandy to the desperate city-wide lockdown, search, and eventual arrest of the suspects associated with the horrific Boston Marathon bombing. We sought to study how well local Sheriff's offices communicate vital information during emergencies and disasters through content analyses of their website homepages. Sheriff's offices have been identified as an integral part of the local emergency preparedness network, but the question of how well these offices communicate to citizens during these events has not been subjected to *any* degree of empirical scrutiny. The website homepages provide an opportunity to investigate a form of communication that is undoubtedly becoming more important within emergency communications networks. Some points of discussion and recommendations for policy emerge from the research.

The degree to which sheriff's offices communicate through their website homepages during emergencies is in many ways similar to LHDs, EMAs and ARC chapters across the nine communication elements scrutinized in the study ($\bar{X} = 48.0$, 45.9, 49.7, 45.6, respectively) (see Fallon et al., 2011; Schmalzried et al., 2011, 2012). The relative absence of substantial variation in the degree to which these different types of agencies exhibit the nine critical communication elements should not be surprising given that *all* of these types of agencies have been identified as key players within the local emergency preparedness network that share the responsibility to effectively communicate critical information during emergencies and disasters.

The research did, however, identify some key differences among these types of agencies in terms of the nine communication elements. For example, sheriff's offices' website homepages are more likely to list the name of the agency's top executive (88.5%) than are LHDs (41.1%), EMAs (64.7%) and local ARC chapters (2.2%). The office of the sheriff is subject to a popular vote of the people, unlike the executive and administrative positions of local government health departments and EMA whose top executives are appointed civil servants. Likewise, the top executives of local ARC chapters are hired by a local board. The fact that sheriff's websites more commonly identify the name of the organization's top executive should be viewed as a consequence of the office's inherently political nature, as well as yet another indication of the sheriff's unique role within the realms of both local law enforcement and emergency preparedness. Popularly elected sheriffs are likely to prominently and clearly identify themselves on the website to maintain public name recognition and bolster bids for re-election. The website homepage provides unique opportunities to accomplish these and other goals irrespective of any current emergency or disaster.

On the other hand, sheriff's offices were much less likely to provide links to emergency preparedness information (6.5%) than were the other types of emergency services agencies, including LHAs (49.4%), EMAs (15.1%), and local ARC chapters (32%). This finding seems to suggest a potential disconnect between scholars and others who analyze the operation of local emergency response networks and the perceptions of local sheriffs in regard to their priorities and role within those networks. The local sheriff has been identified as a key player in emergency response within the empirical literature; but, a majority of sheriffs may view themselves and their organizations as 'crime fighters' rather than 'emergency responders.' This disconnect may be more prevalent in jurisdictions wherein the office of the sheriff is the *only* agency that provides primary law enforcement services. Further study of this can help to more directly measure the perceptions and priorities of local sheriffs in regard to their role within the local emergency response network, and the relative importance of that role vis-à-vis those activities that are more clearly related to law enforcement.

The study also underscored some critical problems for citizens seeking to utilize sheriff's websites during emergencies and disasters that are likely to confuse and/or complicate the gathering of critical information. For example, we note in the section that describes the limitations of our research that the study was complicated by the existence of numerous 'shadow' or nonofficial websites promulgated by candidates for the office of sheriff that were constructed to support upcoming political campaigns. Some of these websites appeared at first glance to be the official website of a local sheriff's office, a situation that is likely to result in considerable confusion by Internet users during ongoing emergencies and disasters. Likewise, close to one-third of the homepages failed to provide links to agency programs or services, and the homepages of only 63.8% of nonmetropolitan sheriff's offices provided such links. This could mean that a large portion of the sheriff's websites act merely as online 'placeholders' providing only some of the reassure critical to citizens during an emergency or disaster. More effective websites that include multiple links to additional programs and services could provide clarity and much-needed additional information to desperate citizens during emergencies and disasters.

One in 11 sheriff's office homepages failed to provide the geographic location of the agency by state. Although such information may seem obvious and relatively unimportant, citizens may not be able to immediately discern whether they are examining the intended website during an emergency or disaster. More than one-half (53.7%) of county names in the USA are duplicates (Fallon et al., 2011). For example, there are 23 local law enforcement agencies named 'Lincoln County Sheriff's Office,' 14 named 'Greene County Sheriff's Office,' and 12 named 'Adams County Sheriff's Office.' Others have confusingly similar names. There is a 'Hot Spring County Sheriff's Office' in Arkansas and a 'Hot Springs County Sheriff's Office' in Wyoming. There are agencies named 'Allegany County Sheriff's Office' in Maryland and New York, 'Alleghany County Sheriff's Office' in North Carolina and Virginia, and 'Allegheny County Sheriff's Office' in Pennsylvania. The duplication and subtle differences in county nomenclature demands that sheriff's offices clearly identify themselves by city and state on the agency's website homepage, and within the related metadata tag keywords relied upon by search engines to locate the intended results for those searching for emergency information through the Internet.

Agency contact information was often lacking from sheriffs' offices website homepages. Roughly one-third (32.7%) listed an agency contact email address, and relatively few (12.7%) provided the ability to sign up on their website for opt-in automatic alerts and emergency notifications. Most sheriff's offices participate in emergency 9–1–1 systems (95% as of year 2007) and their deputies can be dispatched as a result of a call to 9–1–1 (Burch, 2012). So-called reverse 9–1–1 systems are used in many jurisdictions to automatically call telephones in the area with a prerecorded voice message. The problem with these services is that they are limited to calling the universe of directory listed phone numbers having landline telephone service within a specific jurisdiction, as well other phone numbers — including cell phone and voice over internet protocol (VoIP) phone numbers — on an opt-in basis. As consumers drop traditional landlines in favor of cellular and VoIP phone services, counties and cities are increasingly adding automated emergency alert systems that send text messages to Internet-enabled devices in lieu of dialing phone numbers with a prerecorded voice message. Sheriffs' offices may not, however, be the lead county agency responsible for operating these emergency alert systems in many places and that could be reflected in the findings of the current study.

More generally, many of the sheriff's office websites we examined appeared amateur and failed to instill the confidence necessary to reassure the public during emergency and disaster situations. The fact that a majority of websites (62.5%) failed to display the well-recognized pointed-star badge — less than one-third (29.8%) of sheriff's offices in nonmetropolitan counties displayed a badge logo on their homepage[3] — may be indicative of the lack of graphics-savvy web developers in sheriff's offices more than anything else. Schmalzried et al. (2012) found that most local ARC chapters (95.7%) display the ARC logo on their chapter website homepage. This large disparity can be explained by the fact that the ARC promulgates brand standards on their national organization's website with camera-ready artwork of the copyrighted ARC logo available for download and use by local ARC chapters (see ARC, 2013) whereas sheriff's office logos are uniquely local.

Policy implications

There are some clear policy implications generated from this content analysis study. First, we recommend that the nine communication elements identified in our study be used as a minimal standard for the content of sheriff's office website homepages. Uniform placement of the nine elements within a standardized sheriff's office homepage template should also be considered. Content management systems (CMS) commercially available as well as open source CMS software systems could be utilized by sheriff's offices to create, update, and manage website content without specialized knowledge of computer programming languages. The ease of use of web CMS software systems makes them invaluable especially in local government agencies that might lack in-house web developers and other information technology expertise, such as nonmetropolitan sheriff's offices. Costs are greatly reduced when using a web CMS instead of relying on customizsed computer programming to develop agency websites.

We recommend that any nonofficial website of a sheriff or bona fide candidate for an elected office of sheriff include a disclaimer prominently displayed on its homepage with a link to the relevant sheriff's office website homepage. The problem of these 'shadow' websites identified earlier seems to be exacerbated by the webpage within the www.usacops.com domain name on the Internet. USACOPS® is a commercial website that bills itself 'the nation's law enforcement site' that appears to be an online advertising platform for various banner and text advertisements delivered by one or more ad servers. The existence of websites and URLs associated with this online advertising platform and the 'shadow' websites of those hoping to successfully challenge the sheriff in an upcoming election serves only to confuse citizens searching for information during an emergency or disaster.

Additional research should study the use of social media, such as Facebook and Twitter, in emergency and disaster communications. Facebook is an online social networking service used primarily to connect people with friends and groups of interest. Facebook has been used to organize large groups of people in recent social movements and uprisings in Egypt, Libya, and Syria (Barker, 2013) to disseminate crucial information in disaster responses (Houston, 2013), and by public agencies for routine communications and during emergencies (Desouza & Bhagwatwar, 2012). Public agencies such as LHD, however, are often slow to respond to inquiries posted on their Facebook pages (Fallon & Schmalzried, 2013) and unverified information can cause problems in disaster response during complex emergencies (Barker, 2013).

Twitter is a micro-blogging social networking service that allows users to send and receive short text messages (up to 140 characters) called 'tweets.' Twitter has been used as an effective communication tool to establish situational awareness in social movements and activist communities, such as at the 2010 Toronto G20 protests (Poell, 2013) and during the 'Arab Spring' in 2010–2011 (Murthy, 2013). Twitter has proven to be successful in establishing situational awareness during rapidly changing emergency and disaster scenarios as varied as the 2012 Horsethief Canyon fire in Jackson Hole, Wyoming (Kent & Capello, 2013), during the 2010 Pakistan floods (Murthy & Longwell, 2013) and whenever earthquakes are detected by the US Geological Survey (Desouza & Bhagwatwar, 2012).

At the time of our research study, only 15.3% ($n = 397$) of sheriff's office homepages included a link to an agency's Facebook page, and 7.9% ($n = 204$) included a link to an agency's Twitter address. These and other future forms of online social networking are likely to become prominent features of most if not every emergency response network in the USA. Our findings suggest that many sheriff's offices have difficulty creating and maintaining a quality website homepage that can effectively link citizens and critical information during emergencies and disasters. This is an electronic age in which emergency information must be delivered in the most efficient and inexpensive method possible. Webpages suit this requirement, and while most sheriffs' offices are supportive of webpages their content is often lacking. These challenges are likely to become more complicated as the revolution in online communications and social media advances; and, the venerable office of the county sheriff seeks to redefine itself as a key player within the emergency response network going forward.

Notes

1. Cities in the Commonwealth of Virginia are not in counties and are considered independent cities. The cities of Baltimore, Maryland, St. Louis, Missouri, and Carson City, Nevada, are also independent cities that are separate from counties.
2. The bivariate relationship between the number of full-time sworn personnel employed in a sheriff's office and each of the nine communication elements was not explored because the number of sworn employees as a measure of agency size can be misleading as to sheriff's offices. In many jurisdictions, the sheriff's office provides sworn personnel to work in jails and, sometimes, to provide courtroom security. We instead analyze agency size in terms of (a) the provision or lack of routine patrol services and (b) a binary measure of rurality in metropolitan vs. nonmetropolitan counties.
3. This is a surprising finding because the American sheriff's badge is iconic in that it is different than the badges of most other state and local law enforcement agencies and because it is rooted in deep tradition. The distinctive five-point, six-point, seven-point,

or even eight-point star-shaped badges were first fashioned out of the bottoms of old tin cans collected from garbage dumps by city marshals and county sheriffs in the 1870s across the frontier west and soon became the recognized badge of sheriffs throughout the USA (Virgines, 1966). Most sheriff's offices today incorporate some uniquely local version of the pointed-star logo on their uniform patches and cruiser doors (Claflin, 1997).

References

American Red Cross (ARC). (2013). *American Red Cross brand standards*. Author. Retrieved from http://www.redcross.org/about-us/media-resources/logo/brand-standards

Barker, W. (2013). Complex emergencies. In D. MacGarty & D. Nott (Eds.), *Disaster medicine* (pp. 47–60). London: Springer. Retrieved from http://link.springer.com/10.1007/978-1-4471-4423-6_4

Brown, L. P. (1989). The role of the sheriff. In A. W. Cohen (Ed.), *The future of policing*. Beverly Hills, CA: Sage.

Burch, A. M. (2012). *Sheriffs' offices, 2007 – Statistical tables* (No. NCJ238558). Washington, DC: US Department of Justice, Office of Justice Programs, Bureau of Justice Statistics. Retrieved from http://www.bjs.gov/content/pub/pdf/so07st.pdf

Claflin, J. V. (1997). *Sheriffs' insignia of the United States*. Hinsdale, IL: Author.

Desouza, K. C., & Bhagwatwar, A. (2012). Leveraging technologies in public agencies: The case of the US Census Bureau and the 2010 Census. *Public Administration Review, 72*, 605–614. doi:10.1111/j.1540-6210.2012.02592.x

Drake, R. (2009). The hierarchy of emergency preparedness. In S. Hakim & E. A. Blackstone (Eds.), *Safeguarding homeland security* (pp. 31–40). New York, NY: Springer. Retrieved from http://www.springerlink.com/index/10.1007/978-1-4419-0371-6_3

Falcone, D. N., & Wells, L. E. (1995). The county sheriff as a distinctive policing modality. *American Journal of Police, 14*, 123–149.

Fallon, L. F., & Schmalzried, H. D. (2013). A study on the responsiveness of local health departments that use Facebook. *Journal of Homeland Security and Emergency Management, 10*, 201–208. doi:10.1515/jhsem-2012-0066

Fallon, L. F., Schmalzried, H. D., & Hasan, N. (2011). Communications between local health departments and the public during emergencies: The importance of standardized web sites. *Journal of Public Health Management & Practice, 17*, E1–E6. doi:10.1097/PHH.0b013e3181e31d22

Giblin, M. J., Schafer, J. A., & Burruss, G. W. (2009). Homeland security in the heartland: Risk, preparedness, and organizational capacity. *Criminal Justice Policy Review, 20*, 274–289. doi:10.1177/0887403408323762

Hayes, A. F., & Krippendorff, K. (2007). Answering the call for a standard reliability measure for coding data. *Communication Methods and Measures, 1*, 77–89. doi:10.1080/19312450709336664

Helms, R. (2008). Locally elected sheriffs and money compensation: A quantitative analysis of organizational and environmental contingency explanations. *Criminal Justice Review, 33*, 5–28. doi:10.1177/0734016808315588

Hickman, M. J., & Reaves, B. A. (2006). *Sheriff's offices, 2003* (No. NCJ 211361). Washington, DC: US Department of Justice, Office of Justice Programs, Bureau of Justice Statistics.

Hobbs, J., Kittler, A., Fox, S., Middleton, B., & Bates, D. W. (2004). Communicating health information to an alarmed public facing a threat such as a bioterrorist attack. *Journal of Health Communication, 9*, 67–75. doi:10.1080/10810730490271638

Houston, J. (2013). Priorities in post-disaster management. In D. MacGarty & D. Nott (Eds.), *Disaster medicine* (pp. 21–33). London: Springer. Retrieved from http://link.springer.com/10.1007/978-1-4471-4423-6_2

Kent, J. D., & Capello, H. T. (2013). Spatial patterns and demographic indicators of effective social media content during the Horsethief Canyon fire of 2012. *Cartography and Geographic Information Science, 40*, 78–89. doi:10.1080/15230406.2013.776727

Kim, P., Eng, T. R., Deering, M. J., & Maxfield, A. (1999). Published criteria for evaluating health related web sites: Review. *British Medical Journal, 318*, 647–649. doi:10.1136/bmj.318.7184.647

Krippendorff, K. (2013). *Content analysis: An introduction to its methodology* (3rd ed.). Los Angeles, CA: Sage.

LaFrance, T. C., & Placide, M. (2010). Sheriffs' and police chiefs' leadership and management decisions in the local law enforcement budgetary process: An exploration. *International Journal of Police Science & Management, 12*, 238–255. doi:10.1350/ijps.2010.12.2.168

Liederbach, J., & Frank, J. (2006). Policing the big beat: An observational study of county level patrol and comparisons to local small town and rural officers. *Journal of Crime and Justice, 29*, 21–44. doi:10.1080/0735648X.2006.9721216

McCabe, O. L., Barnett, D. J., Taylor, H. G., & Links, J. M. (2010). Ready, willing, and able: A framework for improving the public health emergency preparedness system. *Disaster Medicine and Public Health Preparedness, 4*, 161–168. doi:10.1001/dmp-v4n2-hcn10003

McKing, A. (2008). *A framework for improving cross-section coordination for emergency preparedness and response: Action steps for public health, law enforcement, the judiciary and corrections*. Washington, DC: US Department of Justice, Office of Justice Programs, Bureau of Justice Assistance.

Murray, J. (2005). Policing terrorism: A threat to community policing or just a shift in priorities? *Police Practice & Research, 6*, 347–361. doi:10.1080/15614260500293986

Murthy, D. (2013). *Twitter: Social communication in the twitter age*. Malden, MA: Polity Press.

Murthy, D., & Longwell, S. A. (2013). Twitter and disasters: The uses of Twitter during the 2010 Pakistan floods. *Information, Communication & Society, 16*, 837–855. doi:10.1080/1369118X.2012.696123

National Sheriff's Association (NSA). (2012). *Institute for Homeland Security*. Retrieved from http://www.sheriffs.org/content/institute-homeland-security

Oliver, W. M. (2009). Policing for homeland security: Policy & research. *Criminal Justice Policy Review, 20*, 253–260. doi:10.1177/0887403409337368

Pelfrey, W. V. (2007). Local law enforcement terrorism prevention efforts: A state level case study. *Journal of Criminal Justice, 35*, 313–321. doi:10.1016/j.jcrimjus.2007.03.007

Pelfrey, W. V. (2009). An exploratory study of local homeland security preparedness: Findings and implications for future assessments. *Criminal Justice Policy Review, 20*, 261–273. doi:10.1177/0887403408330637

Poell, T. (2013). Social media and the transformation of activist communication: Exploring the social media ecology of the 2010 Toronto G20 protests. *Information, Communication & Society*. Advance Online Publication. doi:10.1080/1369118X.2013.812674

Reaves, B. A. (2011). *Census of state and local law enforcement agencies, 2008*. Washington, DC: US Department of Justice, Office of Justice Programs, Bureau of Justice Statistics. Retrieved from http://www.bjs.gov/content/pub/pdf/csllea08.pdf

Riffe, D., Lacy, S., & Fico, F. G. (2005). *Analyzing media messages: Using quantitative content analysis in research* (2nd ed.). Mahwah, NJ: Lawrence Erlbaum Associates.

Schmalzried, H. D., Fallon Jr., L. F., Keller, E., & McHugh, C. (2011). Importance of uniformity in local emergency management agency web sites. *Journal of Homeland Security and Emergency Management, 8*(1), 1–14. doi:10.2202/1547-7355.1936

Schmalzried, H. D., Fleming Fallon Jr., L., & Harper, E. A. (2012). Assessing informational website communications during emergencies and disasters. *International Journal of Nonprofit and Voluntary Sector Marketing, 17*, 199–207. doi:10.1002/nvsm.1423

Smith, A. (2012). *Smartphone ownership*. Washington, DC: Pew Internet Project. Retrieved from http://pewinternet.org/~/media//Files/Reports/2012/Smartphone%20ownership%202012.pdf

Strandberg, K. (2004). Sheriff's emergency response teams: More than SWAT. *Law Enforcement Technology, 31*, 8–12.

Struckhoff, D. R., & Scott, R. (2003). *The American sheriff* (2nd ed.). University Park, IL: JRI.

Tan, G. W., & Wei, K. K. (2006). An empirical study of web browsing behaviour: Towards an effective website design. *Electronic Commerce Research and Applications, 5*, 261–271. doi:10.1016/j.elerap.2006.04.007

US Census Bureau. (2012). *Computer and internet use in the United States: 2010*. Washington, DC: US Department of Commerce, US Census Bureau. Retrieved from http://www.census.gov/hhes/computer/publications/2010.html

US Department of Agriculture. (2003). *Measuring rurality: Rural-urban continuum codes*. [Computer file]. Washington, DC: US Department of Agriculture, Economic Research Service. Retrieved from http://www.ers.usda.gov/briefing/rurality/ruralurbcon/

US Department of Justice. (2008). *Census of state and local enforcement agencies (CSLLEA)*. [ICPSR27681-v1 data set]. Ann Arbor, MI: Inter-university Consortium for Political and Social Research [distributor]. Retrieved August 3, 2011. doi:10.3886/ICPSR27681.v1

Virgines, G. E. (1966). Badges of law and order. *The westerners brand book, 23*, 49–56.

Wholey, D. R., Gregg, W., & Moscovice, I. (2009). Public health systems: A social networks perspective. *Health Services Research, 44*, 1842–1862. doi:10.1111/j.1475-6773.2009.01011.x

Yen, B. P.-C. (2007). The design and evaluation of accessibility on web navigation. *Decision Support Systems, 42*, 2219–2235. doi:10.1016/j.dss.2006.07.002

Yeung, W. L., & Lu, M.-T. (2004). Gaining competitive advantages through a functionality grid for website evaluation. *Journal of Computer Information Systems, 44*, 67–77.

Exploring gender differences in constellations of problem behaviors and associated health-related factors during adolescence

Kristina K. Childs

Department of Criminal Justice, University of Central Florida, Orlando, FL 32816, USA

Using data from the National Longitudinal Study of Adolescent Health (Add Health), this study expands on previous research on adolescent problem behavior by (1) examining gender differences in patterns or 'subgroups' of adolescents based on self-reported problem behaviors and (2) identifying differences in health-related factors including service utilization, physical and mental health, and violent victimization across the identified gender-specific subgroups. The data used in this study were taken from Wave 2 of the National Longitudinal Study of Adolescent Health (Add Health) data and includes respondents under the age of 18 ($n = 10{,}360$). Based on 16 problem behavior items measuring delinquency, substance use, risky sexual practices, and status offending, latent class analyses identified a 4-class model for the male subsample and a 3-class model for the female subsample. Important differences in health-related factors were observed across the latent classes. However, these differences were fairly consistent for boys and girls. Implications for prevention and intervention strategies, specifically focusing on the intersection of juvenile justice and public health services, are discussed.

Extensive research, spanning several decades, on the correlation among adolescent risk-taking or problem behaviors has been conducted.[1] Overall, these studies suggest that adolescents who report engaging in a specific form of problem behavior (i.e. delinquency) are significantly more likely to report engaging in other problem behaviors (e.g. sexual risk-taking). Traditionally, these studies have relied on factor analytic techniques to assess the dimensionality of adolescent problem behaviors and have provided support for a unidimensional latent construct (Jessor & Jessor, 1977; LeBlanc & Bouthiller, 2003). Based on this body of research, it has been suggested that the tendency to engage in any one form of problem behavior is part of a general syndrome referred to as problem behavior syndrome or general deviance.

Building on this body of research, as well as previous adolescent-focused research on typologies of aggressive behavior (e.g. hostile vs. relational, reactive vs. proactive), disruptive behaviors (e.g. overt vs. covert), and offender subtypes (based on duration of offending, type of offending, onset of offending), a handful of studies have used categorical approaches to study the co-occurrence of risky or problem behaviors among adolescents. These studies typically involve, at a minimum, delinquent behavior, substance use, and sexual activity and identify between three to five subgroups of adolescents (Bartlett, Holditch-Davis, & Belyea, 2005; Basen-Engquist, Edmundson, & Parcel, 1996; Dembo et al., 2011; Massoglia, 2006; Reinke, Herman, Petras, & Ialongo, 2008). For example, Hair, Park, Ling, and Moore (2009) identified four groups using data from the National Longitudinal Survey of Youth. These groups were labeled low-risk, high-risk, 'drinking and unsafe sex,' and 'smoking, unsafe sex, and lack of exercise.' Similarly, using a sample of high school students, Sullivan, Childs, and O'Connell (2010) extracted four subgroups of adolescents: experimenters, abstainers, high risk-low sexually-active, and high risk-diverse behavior. Childs and Sullivan (2013) also identified four classes of adolescents using data from Waves 2 and 3 of the Project on Human Development in Chicago Neighborhoods representing 'low risk/abstainers,' 'experimenters,' 'drug use and delinquency,' and 'high risk/diverse behavior.'

As can be seen, recent evidence suggests that a categorical approach to describing the underlying structure of adolescent problem behaviors can be useful. However, important questions regarding classifications of problem behaviors in adolescence remain. For example, within this body of research, a clear understanding of the gender differences in taxonomies of problem behaviors has received very little attention. This is an important gap in knowledge because empirical evidence has demonstrated gender variations in (1) the type and level of self-reported problem behavior (Centers for Disease Control and Prevention [CDC], 2013; Huizinga & Jakob-Chien, 1998; Mahalik et al., 2013), (2) risk factors for deviant behavior (Daigle, Cullen, & Wright, 2007; Fagan, Van Horn, Hawkins, & Arthur, 2007; Flannery & Vazsonyi, 1994), and (3) responsiveness to prevention and interventions services targeting one or more problem behaviors (DiClemente et al., 2008; Hsieh & Hollister, 2004; Ogden & Hagen, 2009; Stein, Deberard, & Homan, 2012).

It is possible that variations in the underlying structure of problem behaviors may be accounting for some or all of these previously identified differences. If certain problem behaviors tend to coalesce differently among boys and girls, then it is quite likely that gender-specific risk and needs factors, as well as differences in service responsiveness, are associated with these different constellations of behavior. Therefore, this study builds on existing studies that have applied a categorical approach to adolescent problem behavior by examining differences in the structure of these behaviors for boys and girls separately.

At the same time, the link between engagement in problem behavior and general health has recently become a topic of investigation among public health and criminal justice researchers. It has been well documented that behaviors commonly referred to as 'problem behaviors' such as violence, sexual risk-taking, and substance use are also considered 'health-risk' or 'health-impairing' behaviors. Indeed, serious forms of these behaviors are considered important public health problems. Many have also been found to be associated with a range of negative health-related consequences including victimization, system involvement, and poor physical and mental health (Lauritsen, Sampson, & Laub, 1991; Lynskey & Hall, 2000; Newcomb & Bentler, 1998; Pulkkinen, Lyyra, & Kokka, 2009; Thompson, Sims, Kingree, & Windle, 2008).

A number of explanations regarding this association have been proposed. Some researchers have suggested that engagement in deviant behaviors such as delinquency and substance use directly lead to negative health-related consequences (Herrenkohl et al., 2010; Piquero, Sheperd, Shepherd, & Farrington, 2011).

However, evidence to support this claim is rather inconclusive (Junger, Stroebe, & van der Laan, 2001). Personality characteristics, such as risk-seeking, impulsivity, low self-control, and low self-esteem have also been shown to predict engagement in deviant behaviors and poor health-related consequences (de Ridder, Lensvelt-Mulders, Finkenauer, Stok, & Baumeister, 2011; Miller, Barnes, & Beaver, 2011; Moffitt et al., 2011; Trzesniewski et al., 2006). It is commonly argued that one or more of these personality characteristics leads to a 'risk-taking' lifestyle where adolescents are engaging in a variety of socially (e.g. delinquency) and health-related (e.g. exercise, proper nutrition) deviant behaviors. Relatedly, the concept of problem behavior syndrome suggests that engaging in a number of deviant behaviors, spanning multiple social and health-related domains, may be part of a general disposition towards deviance that can have long-lasting consequences. That is, engaging in any one form of deviant behavior is a 'symptom' of a larger 'syndrome' of unconventionality (Jessor & Jessor, 1977). Finally, another possible explanation for the link between adolescent risk behaviors and poor health is related to social factors or 'stressors' such as socioeconomic status. Adolescents who report serious forms of risk-taking behaviors are more likely to come from lower socio-economic conditions which often means these youth are also lacking health insurance, access to services, and other necessary resources to promote good health.

Yet, most studies examining the relationship between problem behaviors and health-related factors focus on one behavior at a time and rarely consider how the co-occurrence of problem behaviors is related to various health-related problems. The few studies that have explored this relationship have suggested that engaging in multiple problem behaviors increases the chances of poor outcomes later in life. For example, Hair et al. (2009) found that engaging in multiple problem behaviors in adolescence had repercussions in early adulthood. Compared to the 'low risk' group, adolescents in the 'high-risk' group were three times more likely to quit school, almost two times more likely to be unemployed, and nine times more likely to be arrested. Similarly, in a study of 1126 10th and 11th graders, Mun, Windle, and Schainker (2008) identified four groups using cluster analysis with centering for males and females. These classes were labeled 'multiproblem high risk,' 'smoking high risk,' 'normative,' and 'low risk.' At age 24, the multiproblem and smoking high risk groups exhibited low educational achievement, poorer physical and mental health, and heavier substance use compared to the other two groups.

Certainly, understanding the long term consequences of engaging in multiple problem behaviors is important. However, exploring how different constellations of problem behaviors simultaneously coincide with other health-related problems is also an important area for public health and juvenile justice researchers to explore. It is likely that the long-term consequences identified by the Mun et al. and Hair et al. studies were occurring much earlier while the adolescents were engaging in the risk-taking behaviors. For instance, Sullivan et al. (2010) found significant differences in victimization rates and mental and physical health measures across the four extracted problem behavior classes found in their study of high school students (i.e. experimenters, abstainers, high risk-low sexually active, and high risk-diverse behavior). As these findings suggest, by identifying the nature and timing of the relationship among multiple problem behaviors and health-related factors, prevention services that are able to target multiple behavioral, psychosocial, and health-related domains can be developed to curtail the long term, multidimensional consequences identified by previous studies (Hair et al., 2009; Mun et al., 2008).

According to the Risk-Needs-Responsivity (RNR) model, the most effective strategy for reducing poor behavior is to identify each individual's risk for future behavior (risk), assess the multidimensional needs of each individual (needs), and tailor services (responsivity) to the individual's risk and needs (Andrews, Bonta, & Hoge, 1990). The physical and mental health deficits associated with engagement in problem behaviors represent both risk and need, and therefore, should be considered a key element when developing holistic, multi-dimensional programs. Identifying how variations in the co-occurrence of problem behaviors are differentially related to additional health-related factors, and whether gender differences exist, can help identify where linkages can be made between public health services and juvenile justice interventions. For example, the public health approach focuses on primary prevention, or prevention in the first instance, prior to developing serious problem behavior. Typically, primary prevention strategies are also universal in scope, instead of focusing on specific domains of risk. Thus, primary prevention involves identifying and targeting the root causes of poor or unhealthy behavior, which is consistent with the RNR principles that are being adopted by juvenile justice agencies around the country. Therefore, this study seeks to expand on previous research on adolescent problem behavior by (1) examining patterns or 'subgroups' of adolescents based on self-reported problem behaviors among boys and girls separately and (2) identifying differences in health-related factors such as service utilization, physical and mental health, and violent victimization across the identified gender-specific subgroups.

Methods

Sample

Data from the National Longitudinal Study of Adolescent Health (Add Health), a nationally representative study of more than 20,000 adolescents, was used in the current analyses. Add Health used a multi-stage stratified sampling design to select study respondents from 132 middle and high schools from eighty communities across the USA. The first wave was collected in 1994–1995 when the study respondents were in grades 7–12 (for details on the design of the Add Health data, please see Harris et al., 2009). To date, four waves of data have been collected. Across the four waves, the broader Add Health study has included a number of data collection programs including in-school surveys, parent surveys, school administrator surveys, and in-home interviews.

The current study uses data from all adolescents that participated in the in-home interview at Wave 2 ($N = 14,738$, ages 11–22 years). Interviews were conducted in 1996 (April through August). Given that the focus of the current study is adolescent risk-behavior, the sample was limited to respondents under the age of 18 (approximately 24% of the sample was 18 or older). The reason for excluding respondents 18 years of age or older is that some behaviors that may be considered 'risky' to a 14 or 15 years old, may not be considered 'risky' (e.g. sexual activity) or may not be applicable (e.g. skipping school) to a 20 year old. Given the complexity of the Add Health study design, sampling weights were applied to yield national population estimates. Therefore, cases that were missing valid weight components were also excluded from the analyses ($n = 881$, 7.8% of the respondents that were under the age of 18) (see Chantala & Tabor, 2010). These exclusions yielded a final sample size of 10,360 adolescents that were under the age of 18 at the time of the Wave 2 interview.

The final sample used in the analysis was broken down into two gender-specific subsamples. The male subsample included 4924 boys ages 11–17. The average age of the respondents was 15.6 (SD = 1.2). The female subsample included 5436 girls ages 11–17. The average age of the female subsample was 15.5 (SD = 1.2).

Variables

Problem behavior items

Sixteen risk behavior items were included in the latent class analysis (LCA). The selection of these items was based on prior research on risk behavior subgroups among adolescents and the distribution of the items.[2] Violent behavior was measured with two items: how often, in the past year, did you 'take part in a fight where a group of friends was against another group of friends' and 'get into a serious physical fight.' Response categories were measured on an ordinal scale ranging from never to five or more times. Approximately 80% of the sample answered 'never' to both questions. Two dichotomous items measuring previous driving while drunk (91% responded 'no' to driving drunk) and selling drugs (93% reported 'never' to selling drugs) in the past year were also included. Two composite measures were created for property and public disorder offenses. Property offending consisted of five Likert items measuring how many times in the past year each respondent stole something worth more than $50, stole something worth less than $50, went into a house or building to steal something, took something from a store without paying for it, and drove a car without the owner's permission. Response categories were measured on an ordinal scale ranging from never to five or more times. All five items were summed to create an overall property offending index ($\alpha = .74$, factor loadings range from .46–.83, eigenvalue = 2.58). The average for property offending was .83 (SD = 1.88). Public disorder offending was measured with three items: past year involvement in graffiti, deliberately damaging property, and acting loud, rowdy, or unruly in a public place ($\alpha = .70$, factor loadings range from .67–.85, eigenvalue = 1.78). The average of the public disorder measure was .92 (SD = 1.42).

Four items measuring past year status offending were also included. Staying out all night without permission and running away from home were dichotomous variables. Approximately 6% of the sample reported running away from home at least once and 13% reported staying out without parental permission. The number of times a respondent reported skipping school (in the current or previous school year) was recoded into an ordinal scale including six categories ranging from 'not in school' or 'never' to 'more than 11 times.' Four percent of the sample was not enrolled in school at the time of the interview, 70% reported never skipping school, and 3% reported skipping school more than eleven times in the past year. One final item measuring the number of times each respondent lied to a parent/guardian was included. Fifty-two percent of the sample reported never lying to a parent/guardian and 9% reported lying to a parent/guardian five or more times in the past year.

Four substance use items measuring use of alcohol, cigarettes, marijuana, and other, more serious forms of drugs were included in the analysis. Alcohol use was measured by asking respondents how many days, in the past year, he or she got drunk or high on alcohol. Responses were measured on an ordinal scale ranging from 'never' to 'almost everyday/everyday.' Seventy-three percent of the sample reported 'never' getting drunk or high on alcohol. Two items asking respondents to report the number of times in the past 30 days he/she smoked cigarettes and used marijuana were included. The number of times each respondent reported smoking cigarettes was recoded into an ordinal scale ranging from 'never' to everyday. Sixty-nine percent of the sample reported never smoking cigarettes and 10% reported smoking cigarettes daily. Similarly, the number of times each respondent reported using marijuana in the past 30 days was also recoded to an ordinal scale ranging from never to more than 30 times. Seventy-five percent of the sample reported never smoking marijuana in the past 30 days and 5% reported smoking marijuana more than thirty times. Due to the low number of respondents that reported using other forms of substances (i.e. cocaine, inhalants, LSD, PCP, ecstasy, mushrooms, speed, ice, heroin, or prescription pills without a doctor's note), this variable was recoded into a dichotomous variable representing no use or used one or more times. Six percent of the sample reported using other, more serious forms of substances in the past 30 days.

Two additional items measuring the number of sexual partners and use of birth control were included in the analyses. Due to the small proportion of respondents that reported more than five partners, responses to this item were truncated at five to represent five or more partners. Eighty-two percent of the sample reported zero partners and 4% of the sample reported five or more partners. History of unprotected sexual intercourse was coded into three categories representing never had sex, always used birth control, or engaged in unprotected sex at least once in the past year. Sixty-two percent of the sample reported never having sex and 16% of the sample reported having unprotected sex at least once.

Health-related factors

Thirteen items across three health-related domains were examined. These domains include physical and mental health, service utilization, and violent victimization. Items measuring general health included three questions asking respondents 'In general, how is your health' (responses ranged from excellent to fair/poor), the number of times per week each respondent exercised (responses ranged from never to five or more times), and the number of times per week he or she played an active sport (responses ranged from never to five or more times). Respondents were also asked 'in the last month, how often did a health or emotional problem cause you to miss a social or recreational activity?' Given the low number of respondents that reported a high frequency, a dichotomous variable was created representing never missed an event (69%) or missed one or more events in the past month (31%). One additional dichotomous item measuring whether or not a respondent 'seriously thought about committing suicide' in the past year was also included. Eleven percent of respondents reported seriously considering suicide at least once.

Service utilization was measured with four items measuring whether or not, in the past year, each respondent had received (1) a routine physical examination (65% said yes), (2) a dental examination (70% said yes), (3) psychological or emotional counseling (9% said yes), and (4) testing for an STD (5% said yes). In addition to these items, one dichotomous question asking respondents whether there had been 'any time over the past year when you thought you should get medical care, but you did not?' was included in the analyses. Nineteen percent of respondents answered 'yes' to this question.

Finally, five items measuring the frequency of violent victimization in the past year were summed to create an overall victimization scale ($\alpha = .70$, factor loadings $= .53–.77$, eigenvalue $= 2.31$). The five items included witnessing someone shoot or stab another person, being threatened with a gun or knife, getting shot, getting cut or stabbed by another person, and getting jumped (responses ranged from 'never' to 'five or more times'). Due to the low number of respondents that reported multiple victimization experiences, this item was recoded into a dichotomous variable representing never experiencing a victimization and experiencing violent victimization one or more times (18% reported one or more violent victimization experiences).

Data analysis

Analyses proceeded through two phases. First, using the sixteen risk behavior items, a series of latent class models were compared to identify the best-fitting model for the female and male subsamples. The LCA models were estimated using complex survey commands in Mplus 6.0 (Muthèn & Muthèn, 1998–2010). LCA estimates a model that extracts latent 'classes' or categories based on patterns in observed indicators. The patterns are hypothesized to be related to some underlying unobserved factor (i.e. class) rather than being causally related (McCutcheon, 2002). Thus, based on the sixteen observed risk behaviors included in this study, identifiable 'classes' of risk behaviors were extracted.

There is no universally-agreed upon method to selecting the best-fitting latent class model. Therefore, a number of fit and classification quality measures were used to determine the most appropriate number of classes. Lower values of the Bayesian Information Criterion (BIC), which is based on the log-likelihood value of the fitted model, suggest a better fitting model (Nylund, Asparouhov, & Muthén, 2007). The Lo–Mendell–Rubin (LMR) test compares the specified 'k' class model to a 'k–1' class model (e.g. five classes vs. four). Lower p-values suggest that the model with the smaller number of classes can be rejected in favor of the one with an additional class (Lo, Mendell, & Rubin, 2001; Nylund et al., 2007). Entropy is a measure of the quality of classification with values ranging from 0 to 1. Values closest to '1' suggest clearer classification (Vermunt & Magidson, 2004). Lastly, the classification table based on class probabilities for the most likely class membership is also an important indicator of model fit. High diagonal values, typically greater than .90, indicate good classification.

Once the best-fitting models were identified, the posterior probabilities of most likely class membership were saved for use throughout the rest of the analyses. Chi-square tests of significance were used to identify bivariate differences in the health-related items across the gender-specific latent classes. Finally, for items that revealed significant bivariate differences across latent classes ($p < .05$), logistic and multinomial logistic regression models were conducted to identify class differences, controlling for age, across the items. For dichotomous items, logistic regression was used; for items with ordinal response categories, multinomial logistic regression was used. Specifically, the odd ratios (OR) were used to compare classes across dichotomous indicators and relative risk ratios (RRR) were used to compare classes across ordinal-level indicators. All regression analyses were conducted using

Stata 12.0. Survey commands were used to adjust for the complexity of Add Health's survey design and to apply sampling weights to yield national population estimates (see Chantala & Tabor, 2010).

Results

Latent class analyses

The initial latent class analyses entailed the specification of a number of latent class models ranging from two to five classes. The results are presented in Table 1. For the male subsample ($n = 4924$), both the four and five class models had comparatively low BIC values and good classification quality represented by the entropy and average latent class probabilities. However, the LMR suggested that the five class model should be rejected in favor of the four class model (LMR = 2352.28, $p = .00$). Therefore, the four-class model was selected as the best fitting model.

For the female subsample ($n = 5436$), the three class model was the best fitting model. A substantial reduction in the BIC value was revealed (compared to the 2-class model) and the LMR test was significant ($p < .001$). In addition, the entropy and average latent class probabilities for most likely class membership indicated acceptable classification. Based on these results, important gender differences in the number of latent classes, based on the sixteen behavioral items, were revealed. The internal structure of the 4-class model for the male subsample is presented in Table 2 and the internal structure of the 3-class model for the female subsample is presented in Table 3.

The four-class solution from the male subsample identified classes that can be loosely labeled: (1) abstainers, (2) sexually active/substance users, (3) experimenters, and (4) high risk/diverse behavior. Abstainers comprised approximately 61% of the male subsample. Relative to the other groups, boys in this group reported low to no engagement in all of the problem behaviors. The second class, labeled 'sexually active/substance users' comprised 19% of the male subsample. Youth assigned to this class showed the highest probabilities of sexual risk-taking and the second highest probabilities of substance use. For example, the conditional probabilities for the boys in this class were .13 for having more than five partners and .34 for having unprotected sexual intercourse at least once in the past year. The boys in this class also had a .15 probability of using marijuana more than 30 times in the past 30 days, .14 probability of using other, more serious forms of substances, a .26

Table 1. Model fit indices for the gender-specific latent class analysis.

	BIC	Entropy	LMR (p)	Classification
Model fit indices for the male subsample (n = 4924)				
2-classes	125549.94	.90	10688.64 (.00)	.95, .98
3-classes	121775.70	.90	4180.82 (.00)	.92, .96, .98
4-classes	**119834.34**	**.92**	**2352.28 (.00)**	**.92, .96, 1.00, .97**
5-classes	118897.51	.92	1350.18 (.30)	.94, .92, .96, .95, 1.00
Model fit indices for the female subsample (n = 5436)				
2-classes	124917.95	.89	11286.53 (.00)	.94, .98
3-classes	**120321.30**	**.90**	**5006.21 (.00)**	**.92, .97, .98**
4-classes	117807.69	.93	2928.10 (.76)	.99, .93, .96, 1.00
5-classes	116914.82	.93	1311.14 (.84)	.95, .93, .96, .91, 1.00

Table 2. Item-level summary of the extracted latent classes for the male subsample ($n = 5361$).

	Abstainers (60.5%) Means/% (SE)	Sexually active/ substance users (19.4%) Means/% (SE)	Experimenters (13.7%) Means/% (SE)	High risk/diverse behavior (6.4%) Means/% (SE)
Public disorder offenses	.53 (.03)	1.25 (.07)	1.89 (.08)	3.50 (.14)
Property offenses	.10 (.01)	.23 (.02)	2.62 (.04)	6.31 (.05)
Physical fight				
Never	.86 (.01)	.53 (.02)	.58 (.02)	.46 (.03)
1–2 times	.13 (.01)	.38 (.02)	.35 (.02)	.32 (.02)
3–4 times	.01 (.00)	.05 (.01)	.05 (.01)	.13 (.02)
5+ times	.00 (.00)	.04 (.01)	.02 (.01)	.09 (.02)
Group fight				
Never	.90 (.01)	.60 (.02)	.62 (.02)	.40 (.04)
1–2 times	.09 (.01)	.28 (.02)	.27 (.02)	.30 (.03)
3–4 times	.01 (.00)	.08 (.01)	.07 (.01)	.14 (.02)
5+ times	.00 (.00)	.04 (.01)	.04 (.01)	.16 (.03)
Sold drugs				
Never	1.00 (.00)	.79 (.02)	.79 (.02)	.55 (.03)
1–2 times	.00 (.00)	.12 (.01)	.10 (.01)	.14 (.02)
3–4 times	.00 (.00)	.03 (.01)	.04 (.01)	.10 (.02)
5+ times	.00 (.00)	.07 (.01)	.07 (.01)	.21 (.02)
Driven drunk				
No	1.00 (.00)	.78 (.02)	.83 (.02)	.66 (.03)
Yes	.00 (.00)	.22 (.02)	.17 (.02)	.34 (.03)
Stay out w/o permission				
No	.95 (.01)	.69 (.02)	.74 (.02)	.68 (.04)
Yes	.05 (.01)	.31 (.02)	.26 (.02)	.33 (.04)
Runaway from home				
No	.99 (.00)	.93 (.01)	.90 (.01)	.80 (.02)
Yes	.01 (.00)	.07 (.01)	.10 (.01)	.20 (.02)
Lied to parent/guardian				
Never	.69 (.01)	.52 (.02)	.30 (.02)	.19 (.03)
1–2 times	.26 (.01)	.29 (.02)	.39 (.02)	.23 (.02)
3–4 times	.04 (.01)	.08 (.01)	.17 (.02)	.16 (.02)
5+ times	.02 (.00)	.12 (.01)	.15 (.02)	.42 (.03)
Skipped school				
Not in school	.02 (.00)	.10 (.01)	.05 (.01)	.07 (.02)
Never	.82 (.02)	.44 (.03)	.55 (.04)	.46 (.04)
1–2 times	.10 (.01)	.19 (.01)	.16 (.02)	.19 (.02)
3–5 times	.04 (.00)	.12 (.01)	.12 (.01)	.11 (.02)
6–10 times	.02 (.00)	.08 (.01)	.06 (.01)	.08 (.02)
11+ times	.00 (.00)	.09 (.01)	.05 (.01)	.08 (.02)
Number of sexual partners				
0	.87 (.01)	.55 (.02)	.71 (.02)	.62 (.03)
1	.06 (.01)	.11 (.01)	.08 (.01)	.11 (.02)
2	.02 (.00)	.09 (.01)	.07 (.01)	.07 (.02)
3	.01 (.00)	.08 (.01)	.04 (.01)	.06 (.01)
4	.01 (.00)	.04 (.01)	.03 (.01)	.02 (.01)
5+	.02 (.00)	.13 (.01)	.08 (.01)	.12 (.02)

(*Continued*)

Table 2. (*Continued*).

	Abstainers (60.5%) Means/% (SE)	Sexually active/ substance users (19.4%) Means/% (SE)	Experimenters (13.7%) Means/% (SE)	High risk/diverse behavior (6.4%) Means/% (SE)
Unprotected sex				
Never had sex	.77 (.02)	.28 (.02)	.52 (.04)	.44 (.03)
Always used birth control	.17 (.01)	.38 (.02)	.29 (.02)	.29 (.03)
Unprotected sex at least once	.06 (.01)	.34 (.02)	.20 (.02)	.27 (.03)
Drunk/high on alcohol				
Never	.92 (.01)	.39 (.03)	.58 (.03)	.46 (.03)
1–2 days in the past year	.05 (.01)	.16 (.01)	.12 (.02)	.11 (.02)
Once a month or less	.02 (.01)	.13 (.01)	.11 (.01)	.13 (.02)
2–3 days per month	.00 (.00)	.13 (.01)	.07 (.01)	.10 (.02)
1–2 per week	.01 (.00)	.11 (.01)	.08 (.01)	.11 (.02)
3–5 days per week	.00 (.00)	.04 (.01)	.02 (.01)	.06 (.02)
Every/almost every day	.00 (.00)	.02 (.01)	.02 (.01)	.03 (.01)
Smoked cigarettes				
Never	.87 (.01)	.37 (.03)	.53 (.02)	.41 (.03)
1–2 days	.07 (.01)	.11 (.01)	.12 (.01)	.10 (.02)
3–7 days	.03 (.00)	.11 (.01)	.09 (.01)	.09 (.02)
8–14 days	.01 (.00)	.05 (.01)	.03 (.01)	.04 (.01)
15–21 days	.01 (.00)	.04 (.01)	.05 (.01)	.04 (.01)
22–29 days	.01 (.00)	.06 (.01)	.04 (.01)	.07 (.02)
Everyday	.02 (.00)	.26 (.02)	.13 (.02)	.26 (.02)
Marijuana				
Never	.95 (.01)	.44 (.03)	.59 (.03)	.38 (.03)
1–2 times	.03 (.00)	.11 (.01)	.08 (.01)	.09 (.02)
3–5 times	.01 (.00)	.09 (.01)	.08 (.01)	.09 (.02)
6–10 times	.01 (.00)	.07 (.01)	.06 (.01)	.06 (.01)
11–19 times	.00 (.00)	.07 (.01)	.03 (.01)	.07 (.02)
20–29 times	.00 (.00)	.06 (.01)	.04 (.01)	.06 (.01)
30+ times	.00 (.00)	.15 (.02)	.11 (.01)	.26 (.03)
Other drugs				
No	1.00 (.00)	.86 (.02)	.91 (.02)	.72 (.03)
Yes	.00 (.00)	.14 (.02)	.09 (.02)	.28 (.03)

probability of smoking cigarettes every day for the past 30 days, and a .22 probability of driving drunk. This group also had the lowest probability of never getting drunk (.39) and revealed higher probabilities of not being enrolled in school and skipping school, compared to the 'abstainers' and 'experimenters.' On the other hand, the boys in this class showed relatively low levels of property offending and selling drugs.

The third class, labeled 'experimenters,' captured 14% of the male subsample. While the conditional item probabilities were relatively low for the categories representing 'high' frequency behaviors (e.g. skipped school more than 11 times, gotten

Table 3. Item-level summary of the extracted latent classes for the female subsample ($n = 5880$).

	Abstainers (67.7%) Means/% (SE)	Sexually active/substance users (24.8%) Means/% (SE)	High risk/diverse behavior (7.5%) Means/% (SE)
Public disorder offenses	.49 (.02)	1.10 (.04)	2.63 (.13)
Property offenses	.18 (.01)	.67 (.04)	5.41 (.12)
Physical fight			
Never	.93 (.01)	.73 (.02)	.67 (.03)
1–2 times	.07 (.01)	.24 (.01)	.26 (.02)
3–4 times	.00 (.00)	.03 (.00)	.04 (.01)
5+ times	.00 (.00)	.01 (.00)	.04 (.01)
Group fight			
Never	.92 (.01)	.73 (.02)	.63 (.03)
1–2 times	.08 (.01)	.21 (.01)	.25 (.02)
3–4 times	.00 (.00)	.04 (.01)	.06 (.02)
5+ times	.00 (.00)	.02 (.00)	.06 (.01)
Sold drugs			
Never	1.00 (.00)	.91 (.01)	.76 (.03)
1–2 times	.00 (.00)	.06 (.01)	.10 (.02)
3–4 times	.00 (.00)	.02 (.00)	.07 (.01)
5+ times	.00 (.00)	.01 (.00)	.07 (.01)
Driven drunk			
No	1.00 (.00)	.77 (.02)	.60 (.03)
Yes	.00 (.00)	.23 (.02)	.40 (.03)
Stay out w/o permission			
No	.97 (.00)	.73 (.02)	.69 (.03)
Yes	.03 (.00)	.27 (.02)	.31 (.03)
Runaway from home			
No	.99 (.00)	.84 (.01)	.73 (.03)
Yes	.01 (.00)	.17 (.01)	.27 (.03)
Lied to parent/guardian			
Never	.59 (.01)	.29 (.02)	.16 (.02)
1–2 times	.31 (.01)	.36 (.01)	.27 (.02)
3–4 times	.06 (.01)	.16 (.01)	.18 (.02)
5+ times	.04 (.00)	.20 (.02)	.39 (.03)
Skipped school			
Not in school	.02 (.00)	.09 (.01)	.06 (.01)
Never	.84 (.02)	.46 (.03)	.49 (.03)
1–2 times	.09 (.01)	.20 (.01)	.18 (.02)
3–5 times	.04 (.01)	.14 (.02)	.13 (.02)
6–10 times	.01 (.00)	.06 (.01)	.07 (.01)
11+ times	.01 (.00)	.06 (.01)	.06 (.02)
Number of sexual partners			
0	.96 (.01)	.71 (.01)	.69 (.03)
1	.03 (.00)	.07 (.01)	.07 (.01)
2	.01 (.00)	.07 (.01)	.09 (.02)
3	.00 (.00)	.07 (.01)	.05 (.01)
4	.00 (.00)	.03 (.01)	.03 (.01)
5+	.01 (.00)	.06 (.01)	.08 (.01)
Unprotected sex			
Never had sex	.77 (.02)	.29 (.02)	.43 (.03)
	.15 (.01)	.36 (.02)	.26 (.02)

(*Continued*)

Table 3. (Continued).

	Abstainers (67.7%) Means/% (SE)	Sexually active/substance users (24.8%) Means/% (SE)	High risk/diverse behavior (7.5%) Means/% (SE)
Always used birth control			
Unprotected sex at least once	.09 (.01)	.35 (.02)	.31 (.03)
Drunk/high on alcohol			
Never	.93 (.01)	.37 (.03)	.34 (.04)
1–2 days in the past year	.05 (.01)	.27 (.01)	.22 (.02)
Once a month or less	.01 (.00)	.16 (.02)	.18 (.02)
2–3 days per month	.01 (.00)	.10 (.01)	.11 (.02)
1–2 per week	.00 (.00)	.07 (.01)	.10 (.02)
3–5 days per week	.00 (.00)	.02 (.00)	.04 (.01)
Every/almost every day	.00 (.00)	.01 (.00)	.01 (.01)
Smoked cigarettes			
Never	.87 (.01)	.33 (.03)	.34 (.04)
1–2 days	.06 (.01)	.12 (.01)	.11 (.02)
3–7 days	.03 (.00)	.11 (.01)	.09 (.01)
8–14 days	.01 (.00)	.04 (.01)	.05 (.01)
15–21 days	.01 (.00)	.07 (.01)	.08 (.01)
22–29 days	.01 (.00)	.07 (.01)	.06 (.01)
Everyday	.02 (.00)	.27 (.02)	.28 (.03)
Marijuana			
Never	.96 (.01)	.36 (.03)	.32 (.03)
1–2 times	.03 (.00)	.15 (.01)	.11 (.02)
3–5 times	.01 (.00)	.16 (.01)	.13 (.02)
6–10 times	.00 (.00)	.10 (.01)	.10 (.01)
11–19 times	.00 (.00)	.08 (.01)	.12 (.02)
20–29 times	.00 (.00)	.04 (.01)	.03 (.01)
30+ times	.00 (.00)	.10 (.01)	.18 (.03)
Other drugs			
No	1.00 (.00)	.85 (.01)	.69 (.03)
Yes	.00 (.00)	.15 (.01)	.31 (.03)

drunk 3–5 times per week, number of partners), they were also substantially lower than the abstainers in the 'never' categories. This group also revealed moderately high levels of public disorder, property offenses, and probabilities of violent behavior. Thus, these findings suggest that the boys in this group were 'experimenting' or had a moderate probability of engaging in these behaviors. For example, the conditional item probabilities for marijuana use were .59 for 'never' and .11 for 'more than 30 times,' the conditional item probabilities for unprotected sex were .52 for never having sex and .20 for having unprotected sex at least once in the past year, and the conditional item probabilities for skipping school were .55 for never, .16 for 1–2 times, and .12 for 3–5 times. Thus, this group seemed to be 'dabbling' in most of the problem behaviors included in the analyses.

The 'high risk/diverse behavior group,' comprised 6% of the male subsample. Compared to the other three groups, the boys in this group showed substantially higher average levels of nonviolent delinquency (public disorder = 3.50, property offenses = 6.31) and conditional item probabilities for five or more violent behaviors (.09, .16), driving drunk (.34), selling drugs more than five times in the past year (.21), running away from home (.20), lying to parents more than five times (.42), using marijuana more than 30 times (.26), and using other, more serious forms of substances (.28). The only conditional item probabilities where this group did not show substantially higher item probabilities were for getting drunk, smoking cigarettes, and skipping school. These probabilities, although substantially higher than the 'abstainers' and the 'experimenters,' were similar to the sexually-active/substance using group.

In contrast to the 4-class model for the male subsample, the three-class model for the female subsample identified classes that can be loosely labeled: (1) abstainers, (2) sexually active/substance users, and (3) high risk/diverse risk behavior. 'Abstainers' comprised 68% of the female subsample. The girls in this group showed relatively high probabilities of never engaging in the sixteen problem behaviors included in the analyses. The second class, which comprised 25% of the sample, was labeled the 'sexually active/substance-using' group. This group revealed low to moderate levels of delinquent behaviors, while engaging in higher levels of sexual activity, status offenses, and substance use. Most notably, the girls in this group revealed the highest probabilities of being sexually active (.71) and having unprotected sex in the past year (.35). Conditional item probabilities for never using substances were also substantially lower compared to the 'abstainers.' For example, girls in this class had a .37 probability of never getting drunk in the past year, a .36 probability of not using marijuana, and a .33 probability of not smoking cigarettes in the past month. Conversely, the conditional item probabilities for getting drunk once per month and using marijuana 3–5 times per week were .16 and smoking cigarettes everyday was .27. This group also had a .20 probability of lying to parents more than five times in the past year and a .17 probability of running away from home. Thus, this group reported relatively high rates of sexual risk-taking, substance use, and status offenses, compared to the 'abstainers.'

The third class, which comprised 8% of the female subsample, was labeled 'high risk/diverse behavior.' The major distinction between the behavioral profiles of this class and the 'sexually active/substance using' group is the substantially higher levels of delinquent involvement reported by the 'high risk/diverse behavior' group. Girls in this group also showed higher probabilities of lying to parents, running away from home, staying out without permission, and use of marijuana and other drugs. For instance, the probability of using marijuana more than 30 times in the past month was .18 and the probability of using other, more serious forms of drugs in the past month was .31. In sum, important similarities and differences were revealed across the male and female subsamples. An additional class, representing 'experimentation' in a number of different types of problem behaviors was identified for the boys, but not the girls. However, the characteristics of the other three latent classes were quite similar in both the type and level of engagement in problem behaviors.

Associations among latent classes and health-related items

Preliminary bivariate analyses indicated that a number of the health-related items varied significantly across the latent classes (chi-square tests of significance,

$p < .05$). Generally, these variations seemed to be consistent across the male and female subsamples. Only two items, receiving a physical exam and receiving a dental exam, were not significantly different across the latent classes. This finding was consistent across the male and female subsamples. Thus, these two items were not included in the multivariate analyses.[3]

Male subsample

Table 4 reports the logistic (OR) and multinomial logistic (RRR) regression models, controlling for age, for the male subsample. Six comparisons were conducted so that each class could be compared to the other three classes. As can be seen, a number of important differences in the probability of victimization, health-related behaviors, service utilization, and mental health problems emerged across the latent classes. Five of the six violent victimization odds ratios were significant. Compared to the 'abstainers,' the 'sexually active/substance users' were almost five times more likely, 'experimenters' were two times more likely, and boys in the 'high risk/diverse behavior' group were 7.6 times more likely to experience violent victimization. Similarly, boys in the 'high risk/diverse behavior' class were also significantly more likely to experience violent victimization compared to the 'sexually active/substance users' (OR = 1.22) and the 'experimenters' (OR = 1.95).

Important differences in receipt of psychological counseling and suicidal thoughts were also revealed across the latent classes. In particular, the 'abstainers' were significantly less likely to receive psychological counseling and report suicidal thoughts compared to the other three classes. Interestingly, however, there were not significant differences in psychological counseling or suicidal thoughts between the sexually active substance using and high risk/diverse behavior groups and the experimenters and the high risk/diverse behavior class (OR = 0.84). Only marginal differences in suicidal thoughts were revealed between the 'sexually active/substance users' class and the 'experimenters' class (OR = .84).

Relative to boys in the 'sexually active/substance using' and 'high risk/diverse behavior' groups, 'abstainers' were significantly less likely to report fair or poor health, compared to excellent health. Also, compared to 'abstainers,' the 'sexually-active/substance users' were two times more likely, the 'experimenters' were 1.46 times more likely, and the 'high risk/diverse behavior' group was 3 times more likely to fail to get medical care when needed.

Only modest differences across the other three groups were revealed. One significant distinction between the 'high risk/diverse behavior' group and the 'sexually-active/substance users' and 'experimenters' was the higher probability of experiencing violent victimization for the 'high risk/diverse behavior' group. Interestingly, there were not significant differences in the probability of victimization for 'experimenters' and 'sexually active/substance users.' However, 'experimenters' were somewhat more likely to report suicidal thoughts and substantially more likely to report poor general health.

Female subsample

Table 5 presents the results of the logistic and multinomial regression analyses for the female subsample, controlling for age. Similar to the results for the male

Table 4. Multivariate analyses of the health-related factors and latent class membership controlling for age (male subsample).

	Abstainers→sex/drugs	Abstainers→experimenters	Abstainers→high/diverse	Sex/drugs→high/diverse	Sex/drugs→experimenters	Experimenters→high/diverse
	OR (95% CI)	OR (95% CI)	OR (95% CI)	OR (95% CI)	OR (95% CI)	OR (95% CI)
Violent victimization	4.94 (3.78–6.45)***	1.99 (1.70–2.32)***	7.59 (5.45–10.55)***	1.22 (1.03–1.45)*	.94 (.83–1.07)	1.95 (1.25–3.04)**
Suicidal thoughts	3.23 (2.06–5.06)***	1.39 (1.12–1.72)**	3.23 (1.77–5.88)***	.96 (.72–1.28)	.84 (.72–.98)*	1.63 (.88–3.00)
Received STD test	2.80 (1.26–6.21)*	2.05 (1.35–3.13)**	2.20 (.82–5.90)	.88 (.54–1.46)	1.18 (.95–1.48)	.53 (.19–1.46)
Psychological counseling	3.09 (2.10–4.54)***	1.61 (1.26–2.07)***	2.91 (1.80–4.70)***	.96 (.75–1.23)	.96 (.79–1.16)	1.12 (.60–2.07)
Missed social event	1.41 (1.06–1.87)*	1.13 (.96–1.34)	1.67 (1.10–2.53)*	1.13 (.90–1.42)	.99 (.88–1.10)	1.32 (.83–2.09)
Failed to seek medical care	2.19 (1.67–2.87)***	1.46 (1.23–1.74)***	3.14 (2.23–4.43)***	1.21 (1.01–1.46)*	1.00 (.89–1.12)	1.49 (.97–2.30)
	RRR (95% CI)	RRR (95% CI)	RRR (95% CI)	RRR (95% CI)	RRR (95% CI)	RRR (95% CI)
General health rating[a]						
Very good	1.85 (1.45–2.36)***	1.21 (1.02–1.43)*	1.36 (.88–2.12)	.86 (.69–1.08)	.93 (.84–1.03)	.94 (.57–1.53)
Good	2.79 (2.11–3.70)***	1.36 (1.14–1.61)**	2.02 (1.28–3.18)**	.87 (.67–1.14)	.88 (.77–1.00)	1.11 (.66–1.89)
Fair/poor	4.77 (2.76–8.24)***	.92 (.68–1.24)	3.50 (1.81–6.78)***	.87 (.65–1.16)	.57 (.45–.71)***	4.13 (1.82–9.37)**
Exercise per week[b]						
Not at all	1.47 (.97–2.22)	1.11 (.92–1.34)	.98 (.56–1.71)	.86 (.64–1.15)	.96 (.85–1.10)	.81 (.45–1.46)
1–2 times	1.03 (.75–1.42)	1.08 (.91–1.28)	.84 (.55–1.30)	.92 (.72–1.18)	1.06 (.94–1.19)	.74 (.45–1.22)
3–4 times	1.03 (.77–1.37)	.92 (.76–1.12)	.74 (.46–1.20)	.88 (.66–1.17)	.97 (.84–1.11)	.89 (.50–1.56)
Sports activity per week[b]						
Not at all	1.53 (1.09–2.16)*	1.09 (.87–1.37)	1.06 (.51–2.21)	.84 (.57–1.24)	.93 (.80–1.08)	.90 (.45–1.79)
1–2 times	1.69 (1.24–2.32)**	1.24 (1.04–1.47)*	1.28 (.84–1.95)	.88 (.67–1.15)	.97 (.85–1.11)	.84 (.50–1.41)
3–4 times	1.21 (.90–1.63)	1.01 (.86–1.20)	1.11 (.67–1.85)	.98 (.76–1.28)	.96 (.84–1.11)	1.09 (.62–1.90)

[a]Reference category is excellent. [b]Reference category is five or more times per week. *p < .05. **p < .01. ***p < .001.

Table 5. Multivariate analyses of the health-related factors and latent class membership (female subsample).

	Abstainers→sex/ drugs	Abstainers→high/ diverse	Sex/drugs→high/ diverse
	OR (SE)	OR (SE)	OR (SE)
Violent victimization	3.87 (3.01–4.97)[***]	6.19 (4.21–9.09)[***]	1.24 (1.04–1.48)[*]
Suicidal thoughts	3.08 (2.42–3.93)[***]	4.56 (3.29–6.31)[***]	1.20 (1.01–1.41)[*]
Received STD test	4.53 (3.42–6.00)[***]	5.37 (3.34–8.63)[***]	1.07 (.85–1.36)
Psychological counseling	3.64 (2.74–4.82)[***]	4.35 (3.03–6.24)[***]	1.07 (.86–1.35)
Missed social event	1.87 (1.51–2.31)[***]	2.14 (1.53–2.99)[***]	1.03 (.85–1.24)
Medical care when needed	1.75 (1.27–2.41)[**]	2.50 (1.88–3.32)[***]	1.18 (1.00–1.39)
	RRR (SE)	RRR (SE)	RRR (SE)
General health rating[a]			
Very good	1.60 (1.22–2.11)[**]	1.43 (.93–2.20)	.95 (.75–1.20)
Good	2.67 (2.05–3.48)[***]	2.42 (1.59–3.68)[***]	.96 (.76–1.22)
Fair/poor	3.05 (2.12–4.38)[***]	3.66 (2.06–6.47)[***]	1.09 (.79–1.50)
Exercise per week[b]			
Not at all	1.12 (.80–1.56)	.66 (.40–1.08)	.74 (.56–.98)[*]
1–2 times	1.01 (.80–1.28)	.96 (.64–1.45)	.97 (.78–1.20)
3–4 times	.87 (.69–1.09)	.94 (.67–1.31)	1.02 (.84–1.23)
Sports per Week[b]			
Not at all	.97 (.75–1.26)	1.33 (.80–2.21)	1.14 (.89–1.47)
1–2 times	1.04 (.84–1.30)	1.20 (.71–2.01)	1.05 (.80–1.37)
3–4 times	.77 (.58–1.03)	1.13 (.68–1.89)	1.16 (.89–1.52)

[a]Reference category is excellent. [b]Reference category is five or more times per week.
[*]$p < .05$. [**]$p < .01$. [***]$p < .001$.

subsample, significant distinctions between the 'abstainers' and the other two classes were revealed. Relative to the 'abstainers,' the 'high risk/diverse behavior' group was 6 times more likely to experience violent victimization, 4.6 times more likely to report suicidal thoughts, and 4.4 times more likely to receive psychological counseling. 'Abstainers' were also significantly less likely to miss a social event due to an illness or emotional problem and to report failing to get medical care when needed, relative to the 'high risk/diverse behavior' group. 'Abstainers' were also significantly more likely to report excellent health.

Compared to 'abstainers,' girls in the 'sexually active/substance using' group were 3.9 times more likely to experience violent victimization, 3.1 times more likely to report suicidal thoughts, and 3.6 times more likely to report receiving psychological counseling. They were also more likely to miss a social event due to an illness or emotional problem and fail to get medical care when it was needed. The 'sexually active/substance users' were also significantly less likely to report excellent health (OR = 1.6–3.1) compared to the 'abstainers.' Only three significant differences between the 'sexually active/substance users' and the 'high risk/diverse behavior' group were observed. Specifically, girls in the 'high risk/diverse behavior' group had a higher probability of violent victimization (OR = 1.24) and suicidal thoughts (1.20) while girls in the 'sexually active/substance using' group were more likely to report exercising five times a week compared to never exercising (.74). Overall, these results identified important differences in the probability of violent victimization, service utilization, and suicidal thoughts across the latent classes. However, these differences were relatively similar for the boys and girls included in this study.

Discussion

The goal of this study was to expand on previous studies of adolescent problem behaviors by examining gender differences in the number and characteristics of subgroups of adolescents based on self-reported problem behavior and to explore whether these subgroups differed on a number of additional health-related factors. Using a nationally representative sample of middle and high school students, both similarities and differences were observed. The best fitting model for the male sub-sample identified four latent classes (abstainers, sexually active/substance users, experimenters, and high risk/diverse behavior) and the best fitting model for the female subsample identified three latent classes (abstainers, sexually active/substance users, and high risk/diverse behavior). Important differences in the likelihood of violent victimization, general health, service utilization, and suicidal thoughts were found across the latent classes. For the most part, however, these differences were consistent across the male and female subsamples. A number of prevention and intervention implications can be drawn from these results.

The most apparent gender difference observed was the extraction of the 'experimenters' class in the male subsample. This class accounted for a modest proportion (~15%) of the boys included in the sample. Previous studies that have applied a categorical perspective to samples of adolescents have also identified a similar group (Childs & Sullivan, 2013; Mun et al., 2008; Sullivan et al., 2010). Therefore, it is interesting that when males and females are separated, a similar proportion of the females did not fall into an 'experimental' category. The substantive meaning of the extraction of this group for males, but not females, is not clear. On one hand, experimentation in a range of 'risky' behaviors in adolescence is considered a normal part of adolescence. In fact, Mun et al. (2008, p. 291) argued that '... engagement in some level of risk behavior is part of a statistically normative process that is intertwined with age-appropriate developmental tasks associated with increased autonomy and self-regulation.' On the other hand, compared to abstainers, the experimenters were also at an increased risk for many health-related problems including violent victimization, suicidal thoughts, and poor general health. Thus, these findings imply that experimentation may be an important risk factor for a range of health-related problems that carry the potential for negative consequences later in life.

The concept of relative deviance may also, at least partially, explain the extraction of this class for boys, but not girls (Dembo & Shern, 1982; Kaufman, 1978). Research suggests that adolescent boys are more likely to report experimentation in problem behaviors including alcohol and tobacco use, fighting, and precocious sexual activity (CDC, 2013). Therefore, it is likely that experimentation in problem behaviors is considered more normative to the cultural and social expectations of adolescent boys' behavior. According to this perspective, persons who are more deviant from the norms of their social and cultural setting tend to exhibit more serious behavior problems. Thus, engagement in these behaviors by girls is not as accepted by parents, peers, and other important actors (e.g. teachers, counselors) and therefore may lead to more severe forms of these behaviors. Thus, it is likely that the girls that were engaging in these behaviors tended to fall into the 'sexually active/substance using' or the 'high risk/diverse behavior' group. This would also account for the higher proportion of females in these classes compared to the proportion of the males in the respective classes.

Reification is also an important issue when considering the results of the latent class models. LCA provides a useful heuristic for examining heterogeneity in behavioral items across samples of adolescents (Lanza & Rhoades, 2013). The extraction of latent classes is based on patterns observed in the data and do not suggest the existence of actual types of adolescents.[4] Therefore, it is possible that small subgroups can get overlooked in the latent class analyses. As a result, conclusions regarding the presence or absence of an actual 'experimental' group of females or males must be made with caution. Future research is needed to tease out the importance of this subgroup for males, whether a similar group experiencing similar negative health-related problems exists for females, and the substantive meaning of this group for the development and provision of prevention and intervention services.

Our results also suggest that different constellations of problem behaviors are related to varying degrees of risk for poor physical health, violent victimization, mental health problems, and failing to seek medical care when needed. These preliminary findings highlight the complex relationship among problem behaviors and health-related problems. They also call for additional research to dissect the nature and timing of these associations. Some authors have argued that engagement in risk behavior causes poor health-related outcomes (Hair et al., 2009; Oesterle et al., 2004), others have argued that a bidirectional relationship exists (Auerbach, Tsai, & Abela, 2010; Wilson & Widom, 2010), and many have argued that a common underlying trait or disposition (e.g. low self-control, sensation-seeking) accounts for engagement in problem behaviors, poor lifestyle choices (i.e. health and service utilization), and increases in the likelihood of victimization (Gottfredson & Hirschi, 1990; Jessor & Jessor, 1977; Zuckerman, 1979). Although evaluating these causal explanations was beyond the scope of this study, these findings do provide preliminary evidence of a strong connection between engaging in multiple problem behaviors and physical and psychosocial deficits that should not be ignored. These findings also underscore the importance of future research disentangling the causal mechanisms that account for these associations.

Interestingly, service utilization either did not differ (i.e. physical and dental exam) across the latent classes or was higher (i.e. psychological counseling, STD testing) for the adolescents engaging in multiple problem behaviors. Given the lower levels of suicidal thoughts and sexual activity reported by the 'abstainers,' these findings are not surprising. The link between mental health and engagement in problem behaviors in adolescence has been documented for quite some time (Elliott, Huizinga, & Menard, 1989). Nevertheless, the results do provide promising evidence that youth who engage in high frequencies of multiple problem behaviors are accessing services and, at the same time, underscore the importance of integrated strategies that are able to target multiple domains. If adolescents who are at-risk for or are already engaging in multiple problem behaviors are accessing services, the greater the number of risk and need areas that can be targeted in a single setting, the greater the chances of improving the adolescent's health and well-being across multiple domains. Presently, prevention and intervention programs that focus on reducing a single problem behavior are the norm in most child-serving or juvenile justice settings (Office of Juvenile Justice Delinquency Prevention, 2013). It is crucial that these programs involve comprehensive strategies that are based on the RNR principles and target a number of risk and need factors in an integrated fashion. For example, it is widely acknowledged that adolescents are more likely to engage in risky sexual practices while using substances and substance-using adolescents are disproportionately more likely to test STD positive (Hingson, Strunin, Berlin, & Heeren, 1990; Shrier, Emans, Woods, & Durant, 1997). Therefore, sexual health prevention programs represent an effective avenue for lessons on substance use and the associated health-related consequences. This type of program seems to align with the characteristics of 'sexually active/substance users' found in the current study.

A number of limitations of this study should be mentioned. First, although respondents over the age of 18 were excluded from the analyses, the sample still contained a relatively large age range (11–17) spanning different developmental periods. Because engagement in problem behaviors has been shown to vary by age, it may be necessary to examine subgroup differences based on age and gender to fully understand gender differences in the timing and nature of different constellations of problem behaviors. Secondly, since adolescents typically rely on parents or guardians to take them to (and pay for) most services, it is difficult to interpret variations in service utilization without an understanding of the parent's role, income and health insurance, accessibility of community services, and whether respondents were mandated to services (e.g. court-ordered).[5] Finally, although this study focused on the simultaneous relationship between problem behaviors and health-related factors, the use of multiple waves of the Add Health data would have allowed more detailed analyses of gender differences in the nature and timing of these relationships. Identifying the individual, family, and community-level factors that predict membership into each group, for boys and girls separately, would provide a more detailed picture of the specific prevention and intervention needs across each subgroup.

Regardless of these limitations, these findings represent a preliminary step towards understanding gender differences in constellations of problem behaviors. The next, and most critical, step is to identify the risk factors that are related to different constellations of behaviors and whether these are the same for girls and boys. According to the RNR principles, practitioners must be able to identify the specific risks and needs of adolescents, so that effective linkages to treatment can be made. Therefore, a clear understanding of the risk and needs factors that distinguish between different behavioral profiles of adolescents is needed so that prevention and intervention services (i.e. responsiveness) can be tailored to the specific behavioral and health-related problems that these youth are experiencing. Research suggests that intervention programs that are specifically tailored to the risk and needs of particular subgroups of adolescents are the most successful in decreasing high-risk behaviors (Orr, Langefeld, Katz, & Caine, 1996; St. Lawrence et al., 1995). The reason for the effectiveness of tailored intervention programs stems from the acknowledgement that 'adolescents are not a homogeneous population; rather, adolescents are a heterogeneous mosaic of subgroups of different ethnicities/ cultures, behavioral risk characteristics, developmental levels, sexual preferences, and gender differences' (DiClemente et al., 2008, p. 600).

Conclusion

The findings of this study highlight the intersection of juvenile justice and public health. In most jurisdictions across the country, however, this link has been ignored. This is unfortunate because, as Myers and Farrell (2008, p. 1159) point out, 'as youth with increasingly challenging circumstances are channeled into a system ill-equipped to handle their myriad needs, the contemporary juvenile justice system appears to be both overwhelmed and ineffective.' One promising approach to improving juvenile justice system outcomes is to develop partnerships with public health agencies. In particular, a substantial number of adolescents, ranging from low-level offenders to serious, chronic offenders who are engaging in multiple problem behaviors simultaneously come into contact with the front-end of the juvenile justice system (e.g. prevention services, diversion programs, intake screening centers). This stage of the system can serve as an effective avenue for collaboration among juvenile justice and public health agencies. Not only could such collaboration increase the number of services that would be available to youth, it would also increase the scope of risk and need domains that could be targeted through screening and assessment procedures and the development of holistic, multi-faceted treatment plans. This argument aligns with the RNR principles that are becoming adopted by juvenile and criminal justice agencies across the county. By extending the RNR principles beyond criminogenic risk and needs and addressing risk and needs factors across multiple domains, the ability to build resiliency and to avoid costly, negative outcomes will be substantially enhanced.

Acknowledgement

This research uses data from Add Health, a program project directed by Kathleen Mullan Harris and designed by J. Richard Udry, Peter S. Bearman, and Kathleen Mullan Harris at the University of North Carolina at Chapel Hill, and funded by grant P01-HD31921 from the Eunice Kennedy Shriver National Institute of Child Health and Human Development, with cooperative funding from 23 other federal agencies and foundations. Special acknowledgment is due Ronald R. Rindfuss and Barbara Entwisle for assistance in the original design. Information on how to obtain the Add Health data files is available on the Add Health website (http://www.cpc.unc.edu/addhealth). No direct support was received from grant P01-HD31921 for this analysis.

Notes

1. Throughout this manuscript, problem behavior refers to behaviors that have been socially defined as a problem or as undesirable by the norms of conventional society and usually elicits some kind of social control response (Jessor & Jessor, 1977, p. 33). Problem behaviors, deviant behaviors, and risk-taking behaviors are often used interchangeably.
2. Behaviors with less than 5% of the sample reporting engagement in the behavior were excluded (e.g. sex for drugs or money, STD positive).
3. To save space, the results of the bivariate analyses are not presented here. These results are available upon request.
4. The definition of a latent variable implies that it is a hypothetical construct that accounts for associations among observed indicators (Bollen, 2002). Therefore, the latent classes are best regarded as abstractions that help categorize patterns found among the adolescents in the current sample. Variations in observed items and/or characteristics of the sample could change the results of the LCA in substantively meaningful ways.

5. Regardless of these limitations, the service utilization items were an important contribution to the analyses. In order to fully understand the link between constellations of problem behavior and poor health, identifying the services that are commonly utilized/not utilized must be considered.

References

Andrews, D. A., Bonta, J., & Hoge, R. D. (1990). Classification for effective rehabilitation: Rediscovering psychology. *Criminal Justice and Behavior, 17*, 19–52.

Auerbach, R. P., Tsai, B., & Abela, J. R. Z. (2010). Temporal relationships among depressive symptoms, risk behavior engagement, perceived control, and gender in a sample of adolescents. *Journal of Research on Adolescence, 20*, 726–747.

Bartlett, R., Holditch-Davis, D., & Belyea, M. (2005). Clusters of problem behaviors. *Research in Nursing & Health, 28*, 230–239.

Basen-Engquist, K., Edmundson, E. W., & Parcel, G. S. (1996). Structure of health risk behavior among high school students. *Journal of Consulting & Clinical Psychology, 74*, 764–775.

Bollen, K. B. (2002). Latent variables and in psychology and the social sciences. *Annual Review of Psychology, 53*, 605–634.

Centers for Disease Control and Prevention. (2013). *High school youth risk behavior survey data, 2011*. Retrieved from http://apps.nccd.cdc.gov/youthonline

Chantala, K., & Tabor, J. (2010). Strategies to perform a design-based analysis using the Add Health data. Retrieved from http://www.cpc.unc.edu/projects/addhealth/data/guides/weight1.pdf

Childs, K., & Sullivan, C. J. (2013). Investigating the underlying structure and stability of problem behaviors across adolescence. *Criminal Justice & Behavior, 40*, 57–79.

Daigle, L. E., Cullen, F. T., & Wright, J. P. (2007). Gender differences in the predictors of juvenile delinquency. *Youth Violence & Juvenile Justice, 5*, 254–286.

de Ridder, D., Lensvelt-Mulders, G., Finkenauer, C., Stok, F. M., & Baumeister, R. F. (2011). Taking stock of self-control: A meta-analysis of how trait self-control relates to a wide range of behaviors. *Personality and Social Psychology Review, 16*, 76–99.

Dembo, R., Briones-Robinson, R., Ungaro, R., Karas, L., Gulledge, L., Greenbaum, P. E., … Belenko, S. (2011). Problem profiles of at-risk youth in two service programs: A multi-group, exploratory latent class analysis. *Criminal Justice & Behavior, 38*, 988–1008.

Dembo, R., & Shern, D. (1982). Relative deviance and the process of drug involvement among inner-city youths. *International Journal of Addictions, 17*, 1373–1399.

DiClemente, R. J., Crittenden, C. P., Rose, E., Sales, J. M., Wingood, G. M., Crosby, R. A., & Salazar, L. F. (2008). Psychosocial predictors of HIV-associated sexual behaviors and the efficacy of prevention interventions in adolescents at-risk for HIV infections: What works and what doesn't work? *Psychosomatic Medicine, 70*, 598–605.

Elliott, D. S., Huizinga, D., & Menard, S. (1989). *Multiple problem youth*. New York, NY: Springer.

Fagan, A., Van Horn, M., Hawkins, J., & Arthur, M. (2007). Gender similarities and differences in the association between risk and protective factors and self-reported serious delinquency. *Prevention Science, 8*, 115–124.

Flannery, D. J., & Vazsonyi, A. T. (1994). Ethnic and gender differences in risk for early adolescent substance use. *Journal of Youth & Adolescence, 23*, 195–214.

Gottfredson, M., & Hirschi, T. (1990). *A general theory of crime.* Stanford, CA: Stanford University Press.

Hair, E. C., Park, M. J., Ling, T. J., & Moore, K. A. (2009). Risky behaviors in late adolescence: Co-occurrence, predictors, and consequences. *Journal of Adolescent Health, 45,* 253–261.

Harris, K. M., Halpern, C. T., Whitsel, E., Hussey, J., Tabor, J., Entzel, P., & Udry, J. R. (2009). The national longitudinal study of adolescent health: Research design. Retrieved from http://www.cpc.unc.edu/projects/addhealth/design

Herrenkohl, T. I., Kosterman, R., Mason, W. A., Hawkins, J. D., Mccarty, C. A., & Mccauley, E. (2010). Effects of childhood conduct problems and family adversity on health, health behaviors, and service use in early adulthood: Tests of developmental pathways involving adolescent risk-taking and depression. *Development and Psychopathology, 22,* 655–665.

Hingson, R. W., Strunin, L., Berlin, B. M., & Heeren, T. (1990). Beliefs about AIDS, use of alcohol and drugs, and unprotected sex among Massachusetts Adolescents. *American Journal of Public Health, 80,* 295–299.

Hsieh, S., & Hollister, D. C. (2004). Examining gender differences in adolescent substance abuse behavior: Comparisons and implications for treatment. *Journal of Child & Adolescent Substance Abuse, 13,* 53–70.

Huizinga, D., & Jakob-Chien, C. (1998). The contemporaneous co-occurrence of serious and violent juvenile offender and other problem behaviors. In R. Loeber & D. P. Farrington (Eds.), *Serious and violent juvenile offenders: Risk factors and successful interventions* (pp. 47–67). Thousand Oaks, CA: Sage.

Jessor, R., & Jessor, S. L. (1977). *Problem behavior and psychosocial development: A longitudinal study of youth.* New York, NY: Academic Press.

Junger, M., Stroebe, M., & van der Laan, A. (2001). Delinquency, health behavior, and health. *British Journal of Health Psychology, 6,* 103–120.

Kaufman, R. (1978). The relationship of social class and ethnicity to drug abuse. In D. E. Smith, S. M. Anderson, M. Burton, N. Gottlieb, W. Harney, & T. Chung (Eds.), *A multicultural view of drug abuse* (pp. 158–164). Cambridge, MA: Schenkman.

Lanza, S. T., & Rhoades, B. L. (2013). Latent class analysis: An alternative perspective on subgroup analysis in prevention and treatment. *Prevention Science, 14,* 157–168.

Lauritsen, J. L., Sampson, R. J., & Laub, J. H. (1991). The link between offending and victimization among adolescents. *Criminology, 29,* 265–292.

LeBlanc, M. L., & Bouthillier, C. (2003). A developmental test of the general deviance syndrome with adjudicated girls and boys using hierarchical confirmatory factor analysis. *Criminal Behavior and Mental Health, 13,* 81–105.

Lo, Y., Mendell, N. R., & Rubin, D. B. (2001). Testing the number of components in a normal mixture. *Biometrika, 88,* 767–778.

Lynskey, M., & Hall, W. (2000). The effects of adolescent cannabis use on educational attainment: A review. *Addiction, 95,* 1621–1630.

Mahalik, J. R., Coley, R. L., Lombardi, C. M., Lynch, A. D., Markowitz, A. J., & Jaffee, S. R. (2013). Change in health risk behaviors for males and females from early adolescence through early adulthood. *Health Psychology, 32,* 685–694.

Massoglia, M. (2006). Desistance or displacement? The changing patterns of criminal offending from adolescence to adulthood. *The Journal of Quantitative Criminology, 22,* 215–239.

McCutcheon, A. L. (2002). Basic concepts and procedures in single and multiple group latent class analysis. In J. A. Hagenaars, & A. L. McCutcheon (Eds.), *Applied latent class analysis* (pp. 56–88). Cambridge: Cambridge University Press.

Miller, H. V., Barnes, J. C., & Beaver, K. M. (2011). Self-control and health outcomes in a nationally representative sample. *American Journal of Health Behavior, 35,* 15–27.

Moffitt, T. E., Arseneault, L., Belsky, D., Dickson, N., Hancox, R. J., Harrington, H., ... Caspi, A. (2011). A gradient of childhood self-control predicts health, wealth, and public safety. *PNAS, 108,* 2693–2698.

Mun, E. Y., Windle, M., & Schainker, L. M. (2008). A model-based cluster analysis approach to adolescent problem behaviors and youth adult outcomes. *Development & Psychopathology, 20,* 291–318.

Muthén, B. O., & Muthén, L. K. (1998–2010). *Mplus user's guide* (3rd ed.). Los Angeles, CA: Muthén & Muthén.

Myers, D. M., & Farrell, A. F. (2008). Reclaiming lost opportunities: Applying public health models in juvenile justice. *Children & Youth Services Review, 30*, 1159–1177.

Newcomb, M. D., & Bentler, P. M. (1998). Impact of adolescent drug use and social support on problems of young adults: A longitudinal study. *Journal of Abnormal Psychology, 97*, 64–75.

Nylund, K. L., Asparouhov, T., & Muthén, B. O. (2007). Deciding on the number of classes in latent class analysis and growth mixture modeling: A Monte Carlo simulation study. *Structural Equation Modeling, 14*, 535–569.

Oesterle, S., Hill, K. G., Hawkins, J. D., Guo, J., Catalano, R. F., & Abbott, R. D. (2004). Adolescent heavy episodic drinking trajectories and health in young adulthood. *Journal of Studies on Alcohol, 65*, 204–212.

Office of Juvenile Justice Delinquency Prevention. (2013). *Model programs guide*. Retrieved from http://www.dsgonline.com/mpg2.5/mpg_index.htm

Ogden, T., & Hagen, K. A. (2009). What works for whom? Gender differences in intake characteristics and treatment outcomes following multisystemic therapy. *Journal of Adolescence, 32*, 1425–1435.

Orr, D. P., Langefeld, C. D., Katz, B. P., & Caine, V. A. (1996). Behavioral intervention to increase condom use among high-risk female adolescents. *Journal of Pediatrics, 128*, 288–295.

Piquero, A. R., Shephard, I., Sheperd, J. P., & Farrington, D. P. (2011). Impact of offending trajectories on health: Disability, hospitalization, and death in middle-aged men in the Cambridge Study in Delinquent Development. *Criminal Behavior and Mental Health, 21*, 189–201.

Pulkkinen, L., Lyyra, A. L., & Kokka, K. (2009). Life success of males on nonoffender, adolescence-limited, persistent, and adult-onset antisocial pathways: Follow-up from age 8 to 42. *Aggressive Behavior, 35*, 117–135.

Reinke, W. M., Herman, K. C., Petras, H., & Ialongo, N. S. (2008). Empirically derived subtypes of child academic and behavior problems: Co-occurrence and distal outcomes. *Journal of Abnormal Clinical Psychology, 36*, 759–770.

Shrier, L. A., Emans, S. J., Woods, E. R., & DuRant, R. H. (1997). The associations of sexual risk behaviors and problem drug behaviors in high school students. *Journal of Adolescent Health, 20*, 377–383.

St. Lawrence, J. S., Brasfield, T. L., Jefferson, K. W., Alleyene, E., O'Bannon, R. E., & Shirley, A. (1995). Cognitive-behavioral intervention to reduce African American adolescents' risk for HIV infection. *Journal of Consulting and Clinical Psychology, 63*, 221–237.

Stein, D. M., Deberard, S., & Homan, K. (2012). Predicting success and failure in juvenile drug treatment court: A meta-analytic review. *Journal of Substance Abuse Treatment, 44*, 159–168.

Sullivan, C., Childs, K., & O'Connell, D. (2010). Examination of the presence and implications of adolescent risk behavior subgroups. *Journal of Youth & Adolescence, 35*, 541–562.

Thompson, M. P., Sims, L., Kingree, J. B., & Windle, M. (2008). Longitudinal associations between problem alcohol use and violent victimization in a national sample of adolescents. *Journal of Adolescent Health, 42*, 21–27.

Trzesniewski, K. H., Donnellan, M. B., Moffitt, T. E., Robins, R. W., Poulton, R., & Caspi, A. (2006). Low self-esteem during adolescence predicts poor health, criminal behavior, and limited economic prospects during adulthood. *Developmental Psychology, 42*, 381–390.

Vermunt, J. K., & Magidson, J. (2004). Latent class analysis. In M. Lewis-Beck, A. E. Bryman, & T. F. Liao (Eds.), *The sage encyclopedia of social science research methods* (pp. 549–553). Thousand Oaks, CA: Sage.

Wilson, H. W., & Widom, C. S. (2010). The role of youth problem behaviors in the path from child abuse and neglect to prostitution: A prospective examination. *Journal of Research on Adolescence, 20*, 210–236.

Zuckerman, M. (1979). *Sensation seeking: Beyond the optimal level of arousal*. Hillsdale, NJ: Erlbaum.

The effects of treatment exposure on prison misconduct for female prisoners with substance use, mental health, and co-occurring disorders

Kimberly A. Houser[a], Brandy L. Blasko[b] and Steven Belenko[c]

[a]Department of Criminal Justice, Kutztown University, 365 Old Main, Kutztown, PA 19530, USA; [b]George Mason University, 4087 University Drive, Suite 4100, Fairfax, VA 22030, USA; [c]Department of Criminal Justice, Temple University, 1115 Polett Walk, 5th floor Gladfelter Hall, Philadelphia, PA 19122, USA

Inmates with mental health and co-occurring mental health and substance use disorders present difficult challenges for correctional institutions and treatment providers. The complex nature of co-occurring disorders further exacerbates these difficulties and is associated with poor treatment compliance and increased likelihood of engaging in institutional misconduct. The current study examines whether exposure to prison-based treatment reduces involvement in prison misconduct among a sample of female prison inmates controlling for disorder types (i.e. mental health disorder only, substance use disorder only, and co-occurring mental and substance use disorders). Findings revealed that with exposure of more than 181 days of treatment, the odds of misconduct involvement among females with co-occurring disorders more than doubled compared to receiving no treatment. This finding is at odds with treatment retention literature that suggests that a minimum period of time in treatment is needed to affect post-treatment success. Possible explanations for these findings and policy implications are discussed.

Although women comprise a smaller proportion of the overall correctional population, their average annual population growth rate between 2000 and 2010 was higher than that of their male counterparts (1.7% vs. 1.3%, respectively). More than 111,000 women are under the supervision of correctional authorities in the United States (Carson & Sabol, 2012). Many of the women have mental health concerns, substance use disorders, or co-occurring mental health and substance use disorders (COD) (Bloom, Owen, Covington, & Raeder, 2003; Hills, 2004; James & Glaze, 2006; Jordan, Schlenger, Fairbank, & Cadell, 1996; Mumola & Karberg, 2006).

Approximately 73% of women incarcerated in state prisons meet Diagnostic and Statistical Manual of Mental Disorders (DSM-IV; American Psychiatric Association, 2000) criteria for a mental health diagnosis, 60.2% meet DSM-IV criteria for a diagnosis of substance dependence or abuse (James & Glaze, 2006; Mumola & Karberg, 2006), and 54% for both a mental health and substance use disorder[1] (James & Glaze, 2006). Data also suggest that women with mental health disorders are arrested and incarcerated in numbers that surpass their representation in community populations (Lurigio & Snowden, 2008). The high proportion of female inmates with COD and single disorders has important implications for prison management and inmate adjustment to incarceration (Chandler, Peters, Field, & Juliano-Bult, 2004; Serin, 2005), managing misconduct (Houser, Belenko, & Brennan, 2012), and the provision of effective treatment interventions (Belenko & Peugh, 2005; Peters, Bartoi, & Sherman, 2008; Peters & Hills, 1997). If effective treatment can be delivered in prisons, it could reduce the level of misconduct.

Women with co-occurring disorders in prison

The substantial number of female inmates with COD presents a difficult challenge for prison staff for preserving order and security within correctional institutions (Chandler et al., 2004; Morgan, Flora, Kroner, Mills, & Varghese, 2012; Powell, Holt, & Fondacaro, 1997) and provide adequate services to prepare inmates for release (Serin, 2005). Co-occurring disorders are more complex than singular disorders, presenting greater impairment of life skills, worse treatment outcomes, and impulsive and unpredictable personality characteristics (Chandler et al., 2004). Thus, prison management and treatment policies developed for female inmates with singular disorders (i.e. a mental health disorder or substance-related disorder) are likely not effective for female inmates with CODs.

COD treatment programs should combine mental health and substance abuse interventions tailored to the intricate needs of this population (Lehman, Myers, & Corty, 2000; Whitten, 2004). Treatment providers should target issues of mental illness and substance abuse simultaneously, rather than treating each issue as a separate disorder. But implementing such programs in correctional institutions is challenging, requiring a range of staff members and collaboration between departments (Chandler et al., 2004). When prisons have separate mental health and substance abuse departments, it is difficult for inmates with COD to navigate services and as a result they often receive inconsistent messages about how best to address their needs (Peters, LeVasseur, & Chandler, 2004).

Matching treatment needs and risk to prison programming

Inmates with higher needs have more contacts with prison staff as compared to lower need inmates–they accrue more misconducts (Houser et al., 2012), are recommended for higher dosages of treatment, and seek contact from multiple departments in prisons (e.g. medical, mental health, and education) (Serin, 2005). As compared to male inmates, female inmates on average present with a greater number of service needs requiring attention (National Institute on Drug Abuse [NIDA], 2007; Van Voorhis & Presser, 2001). Langan and Pelissier (2001) found, when comparing female inmates enrolled in treatment programming to males, females presented with more serious patterns of drug use, were more likely to have been raised in homes where drug use was present, and were more likely to have experienced physical and mental health problems. Similarly, compared to those with single disorders, female inmates with COD have higher incarceration rates, commit more violent crimes (Steadman et al., 1998), relapse at higher rates, have higher rates of homelessness, and more infectious diseases, such as HIV and hepatitis

(Ditton, 1999). According to the risk-need-responsivity principles (RNR; Andrews, Bonta, & Hoge, 1990), the criminogenic risks and needs of female inmates with COD must be assessed and targeted by correctional interventions in order to reduce recidivism.

Specific responsivity factors also are important because they can influence how one responds to treatment (Andrews, Bonta et al., 1990; Andrews, Bonta, & Wormith, 2006). While enrolled in treatment, women with COD have an increased likelihood of experiencing negative feelings, such as frustration, because of the difficulty involved with multiple treatment needs. The treatment experience may seem more difficult and they likely struggle with achieving treatment success. Therapeutic relationships could also pose as a challenge. Staff might feel uncomfortable or intimidated by inmates with complex needs (Marshall et al., 2002). Female inmates with CODs are less amenable to treatment and are more likely to avoid contact with staff (Ziedonis & D'Avanzo, 1998). As a result, presenting with both a mental illness and a substance use disorder generally means inmates will be less likely to develop positive relationships with treatment staff. The responsivity portion of the RNR model posits that if the treatment approach responds to an offender's learning ability, is sensitive to the treatment setting, and responds to the therapeutic nature of the offender–client relationship, the program will be more successful in reducing recidivism (Andrews, Bonta et al., 1990). Adhering to the RNR model can reduce offender recidivism by up to 35% (Andrews & Bonta, 2010). Available research also suggests that effective correctional programming will reduce prison misconduct by 25% and contribute to positive outcomes for inmates in the community upon release (Serin, 2005). When prison administrators and staff utilize correctional practices that are grounded in research-based methods – evidenced-based practice (EBP) – prison management, public safety, and the emotional well-being of COD female inmates all have the potential to be enhanced (French & Gendreau, 2006; Rice, Harris, Varney, & Quinsey, 1989; Serin, 2005).

Effective assessment and classification in prisons

The primary goal of prison administrators and staff is to maintain safety and order in the facilities (Cullen, Latessa, Burton, & Lombardo, 1993). Effective inmate assessment and classification are hallmarks to the effective management of prisons (Serin, 2005). Essentially this translates to having the right inmates at the right security level in order to reduce prison misconduct and escapes. Acting out behavior by inmates threatens the physical safety and emotional well-being of both staff and inmates (Adams, 1983; Goetting & Howson, 1986). For inmates, prison misconduct causes loss of privileges and jeopardizes early release from prison (i.e. pre-release, parole, and loss of good time) (Toch, Adams, & Grant, 1989). In addition to safely operating their prisons, prison administrators and staff are also responsible for preparing inmates for safe release to the community (Parent & Barnett, 2002).

The two primary goals of prison administrators and staff are empirically related, in that poor institutional behavior is predictive of higher rates of post-release recidivism (French & Gendreau, 2006; Motiuk, 1991). Research across multiple countries and correctional agencies has been consistent in demonstrating that a primary method to reduce prison misconduct *and* recidivism upon release from prison is through effective correctional programming (Andrews, Zinger, Hoge, & Bonta 1990; French & Gendreau, 2006; Lösel, 1995). Prison administrators can ensure safer institutions and communities by providing correctional programming opportunities consistent with evidence-based practices (Taxman & Belenko, 2012). This includes matching the level and type of treatment with the inmate's disorders and service needs (Belenko & Peugh, 2005; Serin, 2005).

Current study

In this study, we examine whether exposure to treatment reduces misconduct behavior of female inmates with CODs and single disorders. We hypothesize that this will hold true, given available research about the link between treatment retention and misconduct data while incarcerated (Serin, 2005). In addition, we examine if there is a moderating effect on misconduct by treatment exposure for different disorder groups.

Methods

Sample and procedure

Data for the current study were drawn with the cooperation of the Pennsylvania Department of Corrections (PADOC). All data used for this study were routinely collected and maintained electronically by the PADOC. Applications were made and subsequent approvals were obtained from the university's Institutional Review Board and the PADOC's Research Review Committee (RRC). All data were de-identified by the PADOC; inmate numbers and names were removed to ensure confidentiality.

Data were provided for all female state prison inmates incarcerated in the Commonwealth of Pennsylvania admitted between 1 January 2007 and 30 July 2009 ($N = 2279$) who were either currently serving or had served time at one of two female correctional facilities maintained by the PADOC (State Correctional Institution [SCI] at Cambridge Springs and SCI Muncy), or the co-educational boot camp, Quehanna. Because upon arrival to the state prison system the intake diagnostic and classification process takes no less than four to six weeks, this study excluded all inmates who were incarcerated for a period of less than four months, which would have been too short a time for them to receive their permanent placement. This criterion reduced the sample size to 2164 cases.

The Texas Christian University (TCU) Drug Screen II (described below) was the major indicator of substance abuse/dependence used by the PADOC at the time of this study. However, 398 cases were missing TCU Drug Screen II scores and were removed from the sample, reducing the sample to its final size of 1766 cases. Univariate analysis of the final sample revealed some missing data, though no single variable accounted for a large proportion of missing cases. The primary independent variable (i.e. no disorders, mental health disorders, substance use disorders, and CODs) had no missing cases. Comparisons of the total eligible sample (maximum $N = 1766$) with the final sample using the most conservative analytic approach for missing data, listwise deletion ($N = 1470$) were undertaken using one-sample t-tests (Tabachnick & Fidell, 2006). Mean differences were very small, although 4 of 17 mean comparisons were statistically significant (see Table 1). Due to the large sample size and the number of comparisons, some differences were expected (Tabachnick & Fidell, 2006).

Table 1. Descriptive statistics for total sample and final sample using listwise deletion.

Variable (Min, Max)	Total sample			Final sample			Sig.	%	N
	Mean	SD	N	Mean	SD	N			
Independent variable									
Disorder group (0–3)	1.34	.94	1766	1.33	.91	1470			
No disorders								10.8	159
Substance use disorders								19.1	281
Mental health disorders								5.8	85
Co-occurring disorders								64.3	945
Dependent variable							*		
Any misconduct (0–1)	.31	.46	1766	.34	.47	1470			
No misconduct								69.9	1028
Any misconduct								30.1	442
Serious misconduct								17.3	255
Minor misconduct								12.7	187
Control variables									
Incarceration length (4–33)	14.48	7.35	1766	15.97	6.92	1470	***		
Location (0–2)	.48	.58	1766	.54	.597	1470	***		
SCI Muncy								51.1	751
SCI Cambridge springs								43.5	640
Quehanna boot camp								5.4	79
Age (18–79)	36.81	9.87	1766	36.87	9.71	1470			
Race (0–3)	.49	.69	1766	.48	.68	1470			
White								61.4	902
African-American								30.3	446
Hispanic								7.2	106
Other								1.1	16
Marital status (0–1)	.15	.35	1762	.14	.35	1470		14.3	210
Current offense (0–1)	.25	.44	1766	.25	.44	1470			
Violent								25.4	373
Non-violent								74.6	1097
IQ score (60–153)	94.39	14.24	1552	94.90	14.20	1470			
Final grade (4–18)	11.26	1.73	1554	11.29	1.71	1470			
WRAT score (0–135)	83.94	35.58	1549	84.68	33.37	1470			
Criminal subscale (1–10)	4.87	1.97	1619	4.88	1.97	1470			
Seriousness of charge (0–2)	1.55	.72	1766	1.52	.74	1470			
Treatment exposure (0–3)	1.49	1.27	1766	1.73	1.21	1470	***		
None								25.6	377
1–90								14.3	210
91–180								21.5	316
181 +								38.6	567

Notes: Seriousness of misconduct was based on an inmate being charged with a minimum of one serious offense; minor misconduct was based on an inmate receiving no serious misconduct charges. *$p < .05$, ***$p < .001$ (Descriptive statistics are based on the final sample of 1470).

Dependent variable

Misconduct is defined by the PADOC as 'a written report completed in response to a violation of a formal rule or regulation by an inmate in the custody of the Department' (PADOC, 2006, p. 10). Every rule violation receives a formal written misconduct report stating the charge(s) and the facts of the case from the viewpoint of the staff member issuing the misconduct (PADOC, 2008). All charges of misconduct are recorded and maintained in the PADOC's electronic database. Using this database, a dichotomous variable was created for any charge of misconduct (0 = no misconduct, 1 = any misconduct).

Independent variables

Diagnostic Categories

Subjects were classified into four diagnostic categories: (0) no disorders (no mental health disorders or substance abuse/dependence); (1) CODs (any mental health disorder and substance abuse/dependence); (2) mental health disorders but no substance abuse/dependence; and (3) substance abuse/dependence but no mental health disorder. Inmates were diagnosed with mental health disorders by PADOC psychology and psychiatry staff members using DSM-IV-TR (American Psychiatric Association, 2000) criteria. Inmates diagnosed with a mental health disorder are placed on the Department's Mental Health and Mental Retardation Roster (MH/MR Roster).

Substance abuse and dependence were assessed by the PADOC Alcohol and Other Drug (AOD) Department staff using the TCU Drug Screen II. The TCU Drug Screen II is a standardized 15 item screening instrument developed to identify individuals with a history of heavy drug/alcohol use or dependence in the past 12 months (in the case of inmates, the 12 months prior to their incarceration). Scores range from 0 to 9 with a score of 3 or greater indicative of substance dependence (Institute of Behavioral Research, Texas Christian University, 2009; Zajac, 2007). The clinical and diagnostic criteria for substance abuse or dependence in the TCU Drug Screen II are representative of those found in the DSM-IV-TR (American Psychiatric Association, 2000) and the National Institute of Mental Health Diagnostic Interview Schedule (NIMH DISC) (Zajac, 2007). The TCU Drug Screen II is used nationally by criminal justice agencies and has been extensively validated with inmate populations (Broome, Knight, Joe, & Simpson, 1996; Knight, Simpson, & Morey, 2002; Peters, Greenbaum, & Edens, 1998; Shearer & Carter, 1999; Simpson, Knight, & Broome, 1997; Zajac, 2007).

Two criteria were used to form the COD group: (1) any inmate meeting the criteria specified above for a mental health disorder (e.g. placement on the MH/MR roster) *and* (2) clinical evidence of a substance use disorder (TCU Drug Screen II score of 3 or greater). The 'No Disorder' group was the referent group and included inmates not listed on the PADOC MH/MR roster and who scored less than 3 on the TCU Drug Screen II.

Treatment exposure

Because time in treatment may reduce time at risk for committing misconduct, as well as potentially curb misbehavior, this study controlled for time in treatment. Further, evaluation studies examining the time needed to affect post-treatment outcome suggest that a minimum temporal threshold must be met before clients will begin to show favorable outcomes (NIDA, 2007; Taxman, Perdoni, & Harrison, 2007). Because duration in treatment has been found to be an important indicator of post-treatment outcome, retention rates may be a proxy measuring client attributes including therapeutic engagement and compliance with the program. Findings of longitudinal studies suggested a three month threshold is needed before clients begin to show favorable outcomes (see Hubbard, Craddock, Flynn, Anderson, &

Etheridge, 1997; Sells & Simpson, 1980). Because of the strong empirical support for minimum temporal thresholds, we coded treatment exposure as a categorical variable reflecting three month time intervals (0 = no time in treatment; 1 = 1 to 90 days; 2 = 91 to 180 days; and 3 = 181 days or more). Treatment exposure was calculated by subtracting the date of admission to the treatment program from the date of discharge. Treatment exposure for inmates who were still actively participating in treatment at the time of the data run was created by subtracting the date of admission to the program from the date of the data run. The total time in treatment per inmate was summed and converted to days. Due to restrictions of the Health Insurance Portability and Accountability Act (HIPAA), we were unable to obtain specific treatment program information. Inmates may have participated in various programs not limited to substance use or mental health programs. In addition, inmates may have participated in more than one program during their incarceration. Therefore, time in treatment included all programs that inmates may have participated.

Covariates

The control variables were selected based on empirical research and guided by the importation theory of prison adjustment on individual-level predictors of prison misconduct. Control variables included age, race, grade level completion, intelligence quotient (IQ) score, reading level, and marital status. Age upon the current admission date to DOC was measured as a continuous variable with a range of 18 to 79 years (mean = 37 years of age). Race was coded into four mutually exclusive categories: 0 = White non-Hispanic (N = 902, 61.4%), 1 = African-American non-Hispanic (N = 446, 30.3%), 2 = Hispanic (N = 106, 7.2%), and 3 = Other (N = 16, 1.1%). The 'other' category was originally defined by the PADOC and comprised .7% of the sample. Due to the small number of Native Americans and Asians in the sample comprising less than .5% of the total sample, these cases were merged into the 'Other' category. Grade level was examined in the current study as a continuous variable (range = grades 4 to 18, mean = grade 11). Grades 13–18 represented post-high school education.

IQ scores have a mean of 100 and a standard deviation of 15 with average scores considered between 90 and 109 (Kaufman & Lichtenberger, 2006). IQ scores were based on the Beta-III, a measure of performance IQ, coded as a continuous variable (range = 60–153, mean = 95). The mean IQ score for the sample in the current study resembles those reported in the PADOC's Corrections Education Outcome Study with a mean of between 92 and 94 for their comparison groups (Smith, 2005).

The current research study also controlled for the reading level of inmates using scores from the Wide Range Achievement Test – Revised (WRAT-R). The WRAT-R is a commonly used screening instrument for screening learning disabilities (Kareken, Gur, & Saykin, 1995; Witt, 1986). The reading component of the WRAT-R converts scores to grade level equivalents. These scores were coded as a continuous variable and ranged from illiterate to first year college with a mean reading level of eighth grade. The mean reading level for the sample in the current study is similar to that found in previous studies of PADOC inmates, with a mean between eighth and ninth grade reading level (Smith, 2005).

Criminal history was measured using the Criminal History Subscale of the Level of Service Inventory – Revised (LSI-R; Andrews & Bonta, 1995), which is a 54 item actuarial classification instrument designed to assess criminogenic risk and need (Flores, Lowenkamp, Smith, & Latessa, 2006). The LSI-R is a standardized theoretically based instrument and has been empirically validated on diverse samples of offenders (Andrews & Bonta, 1995). The criminal history subscale is one of 10 domains included in the LSI-R (Andrews & Bonta, 1995). The subscale values are: (1) any prior adult convictions? (2) two or more prior convictions? (3) three or more prior convictions? (4) three or more present offenses? (5) arrested under age 16? (6) ever incarcerated upon conviction? (7) escape history from a correctional facility? (8) ever punished for institutional misconduct? (including the number of misconducts), (9) charge laid or probation/parole suspended during prior community supervision? (a charge laid means that there was a probation/parole violation), and (10) official record of assault/violence? Each positive response is given a value of '1', which is then summed to equal the criminal history sub-scale total. Thus, the maximum point value is '10' (Andrews & Bonta, 1995).

This study controlled for the primary custodial institution where the inmate was housed, based on the institution where they were incarcerated the greatest amount of time. This had the effect of removing other institutional locations where the inmate may have been temporarily housed for shorter periods of time for classification, medical, security, or other reasons. The location variable was coded accordingly: 1 = SCI Muncy, 2 = SCI Cambridge Springs, and 3 = Quehanna Boot Camp.

SCI Cambridge Springs is a minimum security facility and typically houses female inmates nearing their release date. SCI Muncy is classified as a close security prison responsible for housing all female inmates incarcerated for capital offenses. Quehanna is a military style motivational boot camp classified as a minimum security facility, housing both men and women. (PADOC, n.d.).

Length of incarceration was measured as a continuous variable in months (range = 4 to 33 months, mean = 15.9 months). To create the length of incarceration variable for inmates already discharged, the date of admission was subtracted from their date of discharge and converted to months. Incarceration length for inmates still actively serving their sentence was created by subtracting their admission date from the date of the data run (21 October 2009) and converted to months.

Analytic strategy

To test the hypothesis proposed in the current study, a series of logistic regression models were estimated. An initial logistic regression was estimated for a dichotomous measure of institutional misconduct to examine the probability of prison misconduct among female inmates with mental illness, CODs, and substance use disorders controlling for predictors empirically related to misconduct and controlling for time in treatment.

We estimated an additional logistic regression model controlling for the interaction between treatment exposure and disorder group to further explore the effects of treatment exposure on misconduct. The purpose of the second model was to determine if the impact of specific disorder types on prison misconduct was moderated by exposure to treatment. The interaction term was a two-way product term (treatment exposure × disorder group). Multicollinearity tests between the components and the interaction terms were within acceptable limits. A cross-tabulation of treatment exposure × disorder group x misconduct involvement was then completed to examine the direction of the interaction effect.

Results

Distribution of the independent and dependent variables

Table 1 provides the distribution of the independent and dependent variables and covariates. A majority of the female inmates were not involved in any form of misconduct (69.9%). Most of the women had both a mental health diagnosis and a substance use disorder (64.3%), 19.1% had a substance use disorder only, 5.8% had been diagnosed with a mental illness, but no substance use problem, and 10.8% did not meet the criteria for a mental health or substance use disorder.

The majority of women who received some form of treatment during the current incarceration received 180 days or more (38.6%). Approximately 14% of the women received between 1 and 90 days of treatment and 21.5% had between 91 and 180 days of programming. At the time of data collection, 25.6% of the sample received no treatment.

Greater than half of the sample was White non-Hispanic (61.4%) with 30.3% African-American non-Hispanic. The average age of the women in the study was 38.6. Only 14% were married at the time of incarceration with a mean education level of eleventh grade. The mean performance IQ was 94.9, which would place most of the inmates in the average intelligence category. Wide Range Achievement Test (WRAT III; Jastak & Wilkinson, 1984) scores showed the average reading level of the sample to be approximately eighth grade. At the time the data were collected for this study, 23.5% of the women had been discharged. The average length of incarceration for the sample was 15.9 months. Twenty-five percent of the sample had at least one violent offense conviction for which they were currently serving time. A majority of the women were primarily housed at SCI Muncy and SCI Cambridge (51.1 and 43.5% respectively) with only 5.4% housed at Quehanna Boot Camp. The average score for the criminal history subscale of the LSI-R was 4.8 (range = 1–10).

Multivariate findings

Results from the first logistic regression analysis (Table 2) showed that relative to women with no disorders, the odds of any prison misconduct were 2.2 times greater for inmates with mental health problems and 2.4 times higher for inmates with CODs. Relative to those with no disorders, women with substance use disorders only were not significantly more or less likely to engage in prison misconduct. Treatment exposure at 1 to 90 days or 91 to 180 days did not influence the likelihood of being charged with a prison rule violation, whereas women who were exposed to a minimum of 181 days were 34% less likely of being involved in a prison infraction.

With regard to the effects of other variables in the analysis, for every additional month an inmate remained incarcerated, their likelihood of being involved in misconduct increased by 11%. Relative to inmates housed at SCI Muncy, women housed at either SCI Cambridge Springs or Quehanna Boot Camp were significantly less likely to be charged with any misconduct (51 and 58%, respectively).

Table 2. Logistic regression of prison misconduct on control and predictor variables.

Variables	B	SE	Exp(B)	95% CI
Control variables				
Incarceration length	.104***	.010	1.110	1.088–1.133
Location (SCI Muncy = Ref.)				
SCI Cambridge	−.710***	.144	.492	.367–.545
Quehanna boot camp	−.864*	.344	.422	.213–.818
Age	−.051***	.008	.950	.937–.965
Married at admission	−.312	.205	.732	.484–1.080
Race/ethnicity (White = Ref.)				
African-American	.661***	.150	1.937	1.435–2.632
Hispanic	.085	.270	1.088	.642–1.837
Other race	1.140*	.571	3.126	.986–8.890
Violent current offense	.195	.155	1.216	.913–1.682
Intelligence quotient score	−.004	.006	.996	.984–1.007
Grade level completed	−.085*	.043	.919	.841–.987
WRAT score	−.002	.003	.998	.993–1.003
Criminal history subscale score	.202***	.036	1.223	1.140–1.314
Predictor variables treatment exposure				
(No treatment = Ref.)				
1–90 days	−.399	.233	.671	.425–1.060
91–180 days	−.094	.196	.910	.630–1.359
181 plus days	−.420*	.182	.657	.463–.946
Disorder type (No disorder = Ref.)				
Co-occurring disorder	.879***	.253	2.408	1.444–3.840
Mental health disorder	.790*	.353	2.204	1.085–4.296
Substance use disorder	.507	.277	1.661	.949–2.781
Constant	−.601	.752	.548	

Notes: $^*p < .05$, $^{**}p < .01$, $^{***}p < .001$; X^2 (19, $N = 1470$) = 331.389***, −2 log likelihood 1466.243; Nagelkerke R^2 .286.

The odds of misconduct decreased with age; for every year older, an inmate was 5% less likely to be involved in misconduct. Regarding other socio-demographic variables, being married at the time of incarceration was not found to be significantly related to an inmate's likelihood of being charged with a prison rule violation, nor was their IQ or reading level. Level of educational achievement was, however, significantly related to prison misconduct; the more education a woman received, the less likely they were to be charged with misconduct. Race was also significantly related to misconduct, with African-American women being 1.9 times more likely to be charged with an infraction compared to White non-Hispanic females.

Findings further revealed that women convicted of a violent offense were neither more nor less likely to be charged with a misconduct compared to women convicted of non-violent offenses. Relative to their criminal history, however, the model shows that with each increase in an inmate's criminal history score, the odds were 1.2 times greater of being charged with misconduct.

The model summarized in Table 3 controlled for the interaction between treatment exposure and disorder group. Findings revealed similar results for the predictors found in the prior model (Table 2). However, when the interaction term (treatment exposure × disorder group) was controlled for in the regression model,

Table 3. Logistic regression of prison misconduct on control and predictor variables controlling for interaction treatment exposure × disorder group.

Variables	B	SE	Exp(B)	95% CI
Incarceration length	.103***	.010	1.108	1.087–1.131
Location (SCI Muncy = Ref.)				
SCI Cambridge springs	−.719***	.143	.487	.385–.539
Quehanna boot camp	−.845*	.343	.430	.217–.833
Age	−.051***	.008	.951	.937–.965
Married at admission	−.301	.204	.740	.491–1.095
Race/ethnicity (White = Ref.)				
African–American	.659***	.155	1.934	1.433–2.627
Hispanic	.074	.270	1.077	.535–1.815
Other race/ethnicities	1.106	.573	3.021	.955–8.699
Violent current offense	.134	.153	1.143	.859–1.571
Intelligence quotient score	−.005	.006	.995	.983–1.007
Grade level completed	−.005*	.043	.918	.840-.986
WRAT score	−.002	.003	.998	.993–1.003
Criminal history score	.196***	.036	1.217	1.135–1.307
Predictor variables				
Disorder groups (No Dis. = Ref.)				
Co-occurring disorders	1.008***	.263	2.739	1.606–4.443
Mental health disorders	1.093**	.368	2.983	1.422–5.972
Substance use disorders	.957**	.325	2.605	1.346–4.789
(Treatment exposure × Disorder group)	−.091**	.035	.913	.853–.978
Constant	−.720	.747	.487	

Notes: *$p<.05$, **$p<.01$, ***$p<.001$; X^2 (17, N=1470) = 330.972***, −2 log likelihood 1466.660; Nagelkerke R^2 .286.

all three independent subgroups reached a level of significance not previously found. Inmates with co-occurring disorders and those with mental illness only had a slight increase in their probability of being involved in prison misconduct compared with the original model (OR = 2.4 and 2.2 vs. OR = 2.7 and 2.9, respectively). Inmates with substance use disorders only were 2.6 times more likely to commit any misconduct compared to inmates with no disorders. The interaction term itself was also significant (OR = .91).

Following up on these findings, a cross-tabulation of treatment exposure x disorder group x misconduct involvement was completed to examine the direction of the interaction effect. Cross-tabulations suggested that inmates with mental health disorders or substance use disorders only who received no treatment were more likely to engage in misconduct. Both of these disorder groups were the least likely to be involved in misconduct at treatment exposures of 1 to 90 days, at which point there was a steady increase in their misconduct involvement from 91 to 180 days. However, at 181 days or more of treatment exposure, both the mental health and substance use disorder groups were less likely to engage in misconduct than they were with no treatment exposure. The more surprising result was among inmates with co-occurring disorders. Similar to the other two disorder subgroups, there was a decrease in misconduct at treatment exposures of between 1 and 90 days. However, the COD group's participation in misconduct continued to rise with increased treatment exposure, and was more than doubled at 180 or more days of treatment when compared to receiving no treatment.

Discussion

Women entering correctional facilities have higher disorder prevalence rates compared with their male counterparts and general population estimates (Bloom et al., 2003; Hills, 2004; James & Glaze, 2006; Mumola & Karberg, 2006) creating treatment, safety and order concerns for correctional institutions (Hildebrand, DeRutter, & Nijman, 2004; Houser et al., 2012; McCorkle, 1995; O'Keefe & Schnell, 2007; Steiner & Wooldredge, 2009; Toch & Adams, 1986; Toch et al., 1989). Due to the large number of offenders with treatment needs, the criminal justice system has by proxy become the largest provider of substance use and mental health treatment in the United States (American Psychiatric Association, 2004; Gelman, 2007; Human Rights Watch, 2003).

Providing treatment, however, is only the first step toward effective rehabilitation. Initial screening and assessment of the inmate's risks and needs is integral for effective intervention (NIDA, 2006). Failure to effectively match the needs of the inmate with an appropriate treatment design is tantamount to providing no treatment (Andrews, Zinger, et al., 1990). For services to be effective, they must be tailored to the individual and designed to attend to multiple needs (NIDA, 2007).

The current study examined misconduct charges among female prisoners controlling for disorder type (e.g. mental illness only, substance use disorders only, and co-occurring disorders) and exposure to treatment. At the outset, we hypothesized that as exposure to treatment increased, misconduct behavior of female inmates would be reduced regardless of disorder type. Findings of the initial regression model controlling for exposure to treatment revealed that extended periods of exposure of six months or more reduced the odds of the inmate engaging in misconduct by 35% compared to inmates receiving no treatment services.

Results of the second regression model controlling for the interaction of treatment exposure by disorder subgroup revealed an increase in the odds of misconduct involvement for inmates with mental illness only and COD. In addition, when the interaction term was added to the model, women with substance use disorders only reached a level of significance not previously found. Findings of the cross-tabulation to examine the direction of the interaction effect showed women with COD had lower misconduct involvement when exposed to between 1 and 90 days of treatment compared with no treatment. However, the odds of misconduct more than doubled among women who received 181 or more days of treatment compared to receiving no treatment. This is a surprising finding, particularly as retention in treatment has been found to be an important indicator of success (DeLeon, Wexler, & Jainchill, 1982; NIDA, 2006; Simpson, 1979; Simpson, Joe, & Brown, 1997). Research on prison treatment suggests that a minimum temporal threshold must be met before individuals begin showing positive outcomes following release (Bale et al., 1980; DeLeon et al., 1982).

One potential explanation for this increased rate of misconduct with extended periods of treatment exposure for COD inmates may be that they are in treatment programs not properly designed to address the needs of individuals with dual diagnoses. Treatment in correctional institutions is by nature fragmented (Wexler, 2003), more often addressing the offender's substance use disorder needs over their comorbid psychiatric disorders (Edens, Peters, & Hill, 1997). Failure to address and treat psychiatric comorbid disorders among addicted offenders is equivalent to offering no treatment (Substance Abuse and Mental Health Services Administration, 2006a). Therefore, inmates with CODs may be receiving treatment services that do not address their needs and risk and may actually be having iatrogenic effects. We do suggest some caution in drawing conclusions regarding iatrogenic effects since this was a cross-sectional sample and treatment modality was not controlled for in the study.

However, it would not be surprising to find women with CODs in treatment programs that are not designed to meet their particular risks and needs. The heterogeneity of symptoms and overlapping nature of dual disorders complicates the screening and assessment process (NIDA, 2008). Symptoms associated with substance use disorders may mimic mental illness, such as dementia, amnesia, sleep disorders, anxiety, and psychosis (SAMHSA, 2006b). Conversely, signs of mental illness can sometimes be similar to drug withdrawal symptoms.

Further complicating the assessment process is the lack of dual disorder screening instruments (Sacks & Melnick, 2007). Attention has been largely focused on creating drug and alcohol screening and assessment instruments (Swartz, 2004; Wexler, 2003) leaving many inmates with comorbid psychiatric disorders undiagnosed and untreated (Drake, Alterman, & Rosenberg, 1993; McMillan et al., 2008; Peters et al., 2004, 2008). Swartz (2004) suggests that unless an inmate displays overt psychiatric symptoms, they may go through the entire criminal justice process without ever having their comorbid disorder clinically addressed (pp. 21–25).

Access to integrated COD treatment are lacking in the correctional setting. CODs require integrated treatment designs in which both disorders are treated simultaneously using cross-trained and certified professionals familiar with dual disorders (Lehman et al., 2000; Whitten, 2004). Often the mental health and substance use treatment services operate independently within the correctional setting using different interventional approaches and restricting individuals with disorders outside their area of expertise from participation (Wexler, 2003, p. 225). Even if an inmate is placed in both mental and substance use treatment programs, the different philosophical and theoretical approaches of the programs reduce the likelihood of successful treatment outcomes (El-Mallakh, 1998; Mueser, Drake, & Miles, 1997; Wexler, 2003). Limited resources, staff untrained in dual disorders, and space constraints limiting the ability of prisons to segregate offenders with CODs from the general population are additional constraints that limit integrated treatment services in correctional institutions (Peters et al., 2004).

Although this study furthers our understanding of the implications of COD treatment within correctional settings population, some limitations must be addressed. This was a cross-sectional sample of female inmates limited to one geographic location, Pennsylvania. Therefore, caution should be exercised in generalizing these findings on a national scale. On the other hand, there are several benefits to conducting a study in a single state. All inmates included in this research were sentenced under the same State law; they were all assessed using the same procedures, and they were all subject to the same policies of the same state Department of Corrections. Although comparisons of the original sample and the final sample revealed few differences, findings may also not be generalizable to all incarcerated women in the Commonwealth of Pennsylvania.

A second limitation is the use of the TCU Drug Screen II as the single instrument for screening alcohol and /or drug abuse or dependence. Although this screening instrument distinguishes questions by alcohol and drug usage, the current study only had the final TCU Drug Screen II score and therefore was not able to distinguish between drug use disorders and alcohol use disorders or whether an inmate was considered to have problems with both. Therefore, this study was not able to assess if specific substance use disorders were more problematic than others or interacted differently for inmates with COD. Although the TCU Drug Screen II has been extensively validated with inmate populations (Broome et al., 1996; Knight et al., 2002; Peters et al., 1998; Shearer & Carter, 1999; Simpson, Knight, et al., 1997; Zajac, 2007), it is still a self-reported screening instrument. As such, under-reporting or over-reporting of drug use could reduce accuracy of the diagnoses.

Due to restrictions regarding dissemination of confidential personal information under the Health Insurance Portability and Accountability Act of 1996 (HIPAA), several types of information were not available, such as specific medical information for inmates including specific mental health diagnoses, medication usage, type, and dosage. We were also not able to control for specific treatment modality that inmates received or whether an inmate participated in multiple programs. Because we did not have the dates of the misconduct or treatment services, we were not able to determine whether the misconduct(s) occurred prior, during or after treatment participation.

An additional limitation relates to the validity and reliability of officially gathered misconduct data (see Light, 1990 for a full discussion). Future studies should include detailed qualitative examinations of individual misconduct cases to validate the accuracy of official misconduct data. Such an examination was beyond the scope and resources of this study.

Finally, the current study used the PADOC MH/MR Roster as the criteria for a diagnosis of a mental health disorder. Therefore, it was not possible to distinguish if an inmate was placed on the roster for a mental health diagnosis or mental retardation. However, examination of the sample revealed the lowest IQ score to be 60 with only 1.7% of the sample having IQ scores below 70 suggesting possible mild mental retardation. In addition, each inmate in the study who was on the MH/MR roster had a corresponding DSM-IV mental health diagnosis. Therefore, even if an inmate was deemed to have mild mental retardation they were also considered to have a mental health disorder.

Conclusion

This study examined inmate misconduct by specific disorder type controlling for time in treatment. In addition, we examined whether there was a moderating effect on prison misconduct by exposure to treatment for the different disorder types. Findings revealed that all of the disorder groups had fewer misconduct charges with treatment exposure of between 1 and 90 days. Misconduct rose among all disorder types with treatment exposure between 91 and 180 days. However, at more than 6 months of treatment duration, women with CODs showed a marked increase in misconduct at a rate more than double that of COD women who received no treatment.

These findings suggest that inmates with dual disorders may not be receiving treatment services that match their specific risks and needs. The complexity of CODs presents a greater challenge to correctional institutions compared with singular disorders. The interactive nature of comorbid disorders often exacerbates the individual disorders and worsens treatment outcomes (NIDA, 2008) posing a greater risk for behavioral problems within the institution and lowering the chances of successful re-entry in the community. Therefore, it is essential that effective screening and assessment tools for CODs be implemented during the diagnostic and classification period at intake in the correctional institution. Further, it is important to have integrated treatment modalities within the correctional setting in which both disorders are being treated simultaneously by cross-trained staff in the same setting.

Future research is needed to further our understanding of the effective treatment of dual disorders among female inmates. This includes replicating our findings in different samples, examining the effects of different types of treatment on misconduct, studying the assessment process for incoming female inmates, and conducting longitudinal cohort studies of treatment exposure and misconduct among female inmates in different disorder categories. Inmates with CODs require integrated treatment designs not often found in prison settings. Development and testing of such models are needed to advance our understanding of the complexities of CODs and their unique treatment requirements.

Acknowledgments

The opinions in this paper are those of the authors. The authors alone take full responsibility for errors or omissions that may have been made. A preliminary version of this paper was presented at the Annual Meeting of the American Society of Criminology, Chicago, 2012. We extend our thanks to our colleagues, Wayne Welsh, Matthew Hiller, and Gary Zajac for their help with this research.

Note

1. Some scholars have criticized the mental health statistics provided by the Bureau of Justice Statistics as inflated (see Slate, Buffington-Vollum, & Johnson, 2013 for a full discussion).

References

Adams, K. (1983). Former mental patients in a prison and parole system: A study of socially disruptive behavior. *Criminal Justice and Behavior, 10*, 358–384.

American Psychiatric Association. (2000). *Diagnostic statistical manual of mental disorders* (4th ed.). Washington, DC: Text Revision.

American Psychiatric Association. (2004). *Mental illness and the criminal justice system: Redirecting resources toward treatment, not containment.* Arlington, VA: Resource Document.

Andrews, D. A., & Bonta, J. (1995). *The LSI-R: The level of service inventory–revised.* Toronto, ON: Multi-Health Systems.

Andrews, D. A., & Bonta, J. (2010). Rehabilitating criminal justice policy and practice. *Psychology, Public Policy, and Law, 16*, 39–55.

Andrews, D. A., Bonta, J., & Hoge, R. D. (1990). Classification for effective rehabilitation: Rediscovering psychology. *Criminal Justice and Behavior, 17*, 19–52.

Andrews, D. A., Bonta, J., & Wormith, J. S. (2006). The recent past and near future of risk and/or need assessment. *Crime & Delinquency, 52*, 7–27.

Andrews, D. A., Zinger, I., Hoge, R. D., & Bonta, J. (1990). Does correctional treatment work: A clinically relevant and psychologically informed meta-analysis. *Criminology, 28*, 369–404.

Bale, R. N., Van Stone, W. W., Kuldau, J. M., Engelsing, T. M. J., Elashoff, R. M., & Zarcone, V. P. (1980). Therapeutic communities vs. methadone maintenance. A prospective study of narcotic addiction treatment: Design and one year follow-up results. *Archives of General Psychiatry, 37*, 179–193.

Belenko, S., & Peugh, J. (2005). Estimating drug treatment needs among state prison inmates. *Drug and Alcohol Dependence, 77*, 269–281.

Bloom, B., Owen, B., Covington, S., & Raeder, M. (2003). *Gender responsive strategies: Research, practice, and guiding principles for women offenders.* Washington, DC: National Institute of Corrections, US Department of Justice.

Broome, K. M., Knight, K., Joe, G. W., & Simpson, D. D. (1996). Evaluating the drug abusing probationer: Clinical interview versus self-administered assessment. *Criminal Justice and behavior, 23*, 593–606.

Carson, E. A., & Sabol, W. J. (2012). *Prisoners in 2011.* Washington, DC: Bureau of Justice Statistics, US Department of Justice.

Chandler, R. K., Peters, R. H., Field, G., & Juliano-Bult, D. (2004). Challenges in implementing evidence-based treatment practices for co-occurring disorders in the criminal justice system. *Behavioral Sciences and the Law, 22*, 431–448.

Cullen, F. T., Latessa, E. J., Burton, V. S., & Lombardo, L. X. (1993). Correctional orientation of prison wardens: Is the rehabilitative ideal supported? *Criminology, 31*, 69–92.

DeLeon, G., Wexler, H., & Jainchill, N. (1982). The therapeutic community: Success and improvement rates 5 years after treatment. *International Journal of Addictions, 17*, 703–747.

Ditton, P. M. (1999). *Special report mental health and treatment of inmates and probationers.* Washington, DC: US Department of Justice, Bureau of Justice Statistics.

Drake, R. E., Alterman, A. I., & Rosenberg, S. R. (1993). Detection of substance use disorders in severely mentally ill patients. *Community Mental Health Journal, 29*, 175–192.

Edens, J. F., Peters, R. H., & Hills, H. A. (1997). Treating prison inmates with co-occurring disorders: An integrative review of existing programs. *Behavioral Science and Law, 15*, 439–457.

El-Mallakh, P. (1998). Treatment models for clients with co-occurring addictive and mental disorders. *Archives of Psychiatric Nursing, XII*, 71–80.

Flores, A. W., Lowenkamp, C. T., Smith, P., & Latessa, E. (2006). Validating the level of service inventory-revised on a sample of federal probationers. *Federal Probation, 70*, 44–48.

French, S. A., & Gendreau, P. (2006). Reducing prison misconducts: What works! *Criminal Justice and Behavior, 33*, 185–218.

Gelman, D. (2007). Managing inmates with mental health disorders. *Corrections Today, 22*–23.

Goetting, A., & Howson, R. M. (1986). Correlates of prisoner misconduct. *Journal of Quantitative Criminology, 2*, 49–67.

Hildebrand, M., De Ruiter, C., & Nijman, H. (2004). PCL-R psychopathy predicts disruptive behavior among male offenders in a Dutch forensic psychiatric hospital. *Journal of Interpersonal Violence, 19*, 13–29.

Hills, H. (2004). *The special needs of women with co-occurring disorders diverted from the criminal justice system*. Delmar, NY: The National GAINS Center for People with Co-occurring Disorders in Contact with the Justice System.

Houser, K., Belenko, S., & Brennan, P. (2012). The effects of mental health and substance abuse disorders on institutional misconduct among female inmates. *Justice Quarterly, 29*, 799–828.

Hubbard, R. L., Craddock, G. S., Flynn, P. M., Anderson, J., & Etheridge, R. M. (1997). Overview of 1-year follow-up outcomes in the Drug Abuse Treatment Outcome Study (DATOS). *Psychology of Addictive Behaviors, 11*, 261–278.

Human Rights Watch. (2003). *Keep mentally ill out of solitary confinement*. Retrieved June 18, 2000, from http://www.hrw.org

Institute of Behavioral Research, Texas Christian University. (2009). *Correctional residential treatment*. Retrieved October, 20, 2009, from Institute of Behavior Research website: http://www.ibr.tcu.edu/pubs/datacoll/cjforms.html

James, D. J., & Glaze, L. E. (2006). *Mental health problems of prison and jail inmates*. Washington, DC: Bureau of Justice Statistics, US Department of Justice.

Jastak, S., & Wilkinson, G. (1984). *WRAT-R: Wide range achievement test revised administration manual*. Wilmington, DE: Jastak Associates.

Jordan, B. K., Schlenger, W. E., Fairbank, J. A., & Caddell, J. M. (1996). Prevalence of psychiatric disorders among incarcerated women: II. Convicted felons entering prison. *Archives of General Psychiatry, 53*, 513–519.

Kareken, D. A., Gur, R. C., & Saykin, A. J. (1995). Reading on the wide range achievement test-revised and parental education as predictors of IQ: Comparison with the Barona formula. *Archives of Clinical Neuropsychology, 10*, 147–157.

Kaufman, A. S., & Lichtenberger, E. O. (2006). *Assessing adolescent and adult intelligence* (3rd ed.). Hoboken, NJ: John Wiley & Sons Inc.

Knight, K., Simpson, D. D., & Morey, J. T. (2002). *Evaluation of the TCU Drug Screen*. (Pub. No. 196682). Washington, DC: National Institute of Justice, US. Department of Justice.

Langan, N. P., & Pelissier, B. M. (2001). Gender differences among prisoners in drug treatment. *Journal of Substance Abuse, 13*, 291–301.

Lehman, A. F., Myers, C. P., & Corty, E. (2000). Assessment and classification of patients with psychiatric and substance abuse syndromes. *Psychiatric Services, 51*, 1119–1125.

Light, S. (1990). Measurement error in official statistics: Prison rule infraction data. *Federal Probation, 54*, 63–68.

Lösel, F. (1995). The efficacy of correctional treatment: A review and synthesis of meta-evaluations. In J. McGuire (Ed.), *What works: Reducing reoffending: Guidelines from research and practice* (pp. 79–114). Oxford: John Wiley.

Lurigio, A. J., & Snowden, J. (2008). The impact of prison culture on the treatment and control of mentally ill offenders. In J. Byrne, D. Hummer, & F. S. Taxman (Eds.), *Prison violence, prison culture, and offender change* (pp. 164–179). Upper Saddle River, NJ: Allyn and Bacon.

Marshall, W. L., Serran, G. A., Moulden, H., Mulloy, R., Fernandez, Y. M., Mann, R., & Thornton, D. (2002). Therapist features in sexual offender treatment: Their reliable identification and influence in behaviour change. *Clinical Psychology and Psychotherapy, 9*, 395–405.

McCorkle, R. C. (1995). Gender, psychopathology, and institutional behavior: A comparison of male and female mentally ill prison inmates. *Journal of Criminal Justice, 23*, 53–61.

McMillan, G. P., Timken, D. S., Lapidus, J., C'de Baca, J., Lapham, S. C., & McNeal, M. (2008). Underdiagnosis of comorbid mental illness in repeat DUI offenders mandated to treatment. *Journal of Substance Abuse Treatment, 34*, 320–325.

Morgan, R. G., Flora, D. G., Kroner, D. G., Mills, J. F., & Varghese, F. (2012). Treating offenders with mental illness: A research synthesis. *Law and Human Behavior, 36*, 37–50.

Motiuk, L. (1991). *Antecedents and consequences of prison adjustment: A systematic assessment and reassessment approach.* (Unpublished doctoral dissertation, Carleton University).

Mueser, K. T., Drake, R. E., & Miles, K. M. (1997). The course and treatment of substance use disorders in persons with severe mental illness. In L. S. Onken, J. D. Blaine, S. Genser, & A. M. Horton (Eds.), *Treatment of drug dependent individuals with comorbid mental disorders* (NIH Publication No. 97-4172) (pp. 86–109). Washington, DC: US Department of Health and Human Services.

Mumola, C. J., & Karberg, J. C. (2006). *Drug use and dependence, State and Federal prisoners, 2004.* Washington, DC: Bureau of Justice Statistics, US Department of Justice.

National Institute on Drug Abuse (NIDA). (2006). *Treatment for drug abusers in the criminal justice system.* Washington, DC: US Department of Health and Human Services.

National Institute on Drug Abuse (NIDA). (2007). *Understanding drug abuse and addiction: What science says.* Washington, DC: US Department of Health and Human Services.

National Institute on Drug Abuse (NIDA). (2008). *Comorbidity: Addiction and other mental illnesses.* Washington, DC: US Department of Health and Human Services.

O'Keefe, M. L., & Schnell, M. J. (2007). Offenders with mental illness in the correctional system. *Mental Health Issues in the Criminal Justice System, 46*, 81–104.

Parent, D. G., & Barnett, L. (2002). *Transitions from prison to community initiatives.* Washington, DC: National Institute of Corrections.

Pennsylvania Department of Corrections (PADOC). (2006). *Handbook for families and friends of pennsylvania department of corrections prison inmates.* Retrieved September 5, 2009, from the Pennsylvania Department of Corrections website: http://www.cor.state.pa.us/portal/lib/bis/Handbook_for_Families_and_Friends.pdf

Pennsylvania Department of Corrections (PADOC). (2008). *Inmate Discipline.* Retrieved November 2, 2009, from the Pennsylvania Department of Corrections website: http://www.cor.state.pa.us/standards/lib/standards/801_Inmate_Discipline.pdf

Pennsylvania Department of Corrections. (n.d.). *Institutions.* Retrieved September 12, 2009, from the Pennsylvania Department of Corrections website: http://www.portal.state.pa.us/portal/server.pt/community/institutions/5270

Peters, R. H., Bartoi, M. B. G., & Sherman, P. B. (2008). *Screening and assessment of co-occurring disorders in the justice system.* Delmar, NY: CMHS National GAINS Center.

Peters, R. H., Greenbaum, P. E., & Edens, J. F. (1998). Prevalence of *DSM-IV* substance abuse and dependence disorders among prison inmates. *The American Journal of Drug and Alcohol Abuse, 24*, 573–587.

Peters, R. H., & Hills, H. (1997). *Intervention strategies for offenders with co-occurring disorders: What works?* Delmar, NY: National GAINS Center.

Peters, R. H., LeVasseur, M. E., & Chandler, R. K. (2004). Correctional treatment for co-occurring disorders: Results from a national survey. *Behavioral Science and the Law, 22*, 563–584.

Powell, T. A., Holt, J. C., & Fondacaro, K. M. (1997). The prevalence of mental illness among inmates in a rural state. *Law and Human Behavior, 21*, 427–438.

Rice, M. E., Harris, G. T., Varney, G. W., & Quinsey, V. L. (1989). *Violence in institutions: Understanding. prevention, and control.* Toronto: Hans Huber.

Sacks, S., & Melnick, G. (2007). *Brief report: Criminal justice co-occurring disorder screening instrument (CJ-CODSI)*. Washington, DC: National Institute on Drug Abuse, National Institutes of Health.

Sells, S. B., & Simpson, D. D. (1980). The case for drug abuse treatment effectiveness, based on the DARP research program. *British Journal of Addictions, 75*, 117–131.

Serin, R. C. (2005). *Evidence-based practice: Principles for enhancing correctional results in prisons*. Washington, DC: US Department of Justice, National Institute of Corrections.

Shearer, R. A., & Carter, C. R. (1999). Screening and assessing substance abusing offenders: Quantity and quality. *Federal Probation, 63*, 30–34.

Simpson, D. D. (1979). The relation of time spent in drug abuse treatment to post-treatment outcome. *American Journal of Psychiatry, 136*, 1449–1453.

Simpson, D. D., Joe, G. W., & Brown, B. S. (1997). Treatment retention and follow-up outcomes in the Drug Abuse Treatment Outcome Study (DATOS). *Psychology of Addictive Behaviors, 11*, 294–307.

Simpson, D. D., Knight, K., & Broome, K. M. (1997). *TCU/CJ forms manual: TCU drug screen and initial assessment*. Fort Worth, TX: Texas Christian University, Institute of Behavioral Research.

Slate, R. N., Buffington-Vollum, J. K., & Johnson, W. (2013). *The criminalization of mental illness: Crisis and opportunity for the justice system* (2nd ed.). Durham, NC: Carolina Academic Press.

Smith, L. G. (2005). *Pennsylvania department of corrections education outcome study*. Retrieved January 2, 2011, from http://www.portal.state.pa.us/portal/server.pt

Steadman, H. J., Mulvey, E. P., Monohan, J., Robbins, P. C., Appelbaum, P. S., Grisso, T., Roth, L. H., & Silver, E. (1998). Violence by people discharged from acute psychiatric facilities and by others in the same neighborhoods. *Archives of General Psychiatry, 55*, 393–401.

Steiner, B., & Wooldredge, J. (2009). Individual and environmental effects on assaults and nonviolent rule breaking by women in prison. *Journal of Research in Crime and Delinquency, 46*, 437–467.

Substance Abuse and Mental Health Services Administration (SAMHSA). (2006a). *Overarching principles to address the needs of persons with co-occurring disorders*. Washington, DC: Department of Health and Human Services.

Substance Abuse and Mental Health Services Administration (SAMHSA). (2006b). *Definition and terms relating to co-occurring disorders*. Washington, D.C: Department of Health and Human Services.

Swartz, J. A. (2004). Considering psychiatric comorbidities among addicted offenders: A new strategy for client-treatment matching. In K. Knight, & D. Farabee (Eds.), *Treating addicted offenders; a continuum of effective practices* (pp. 21-1–21-13). Kingston, N.J: Civic Research Institute.

Tabachnick, B. G., & Fidell, L. S. (2006). *Using multivariate statistics* (5th ed.). New York, NY: Harper Collins.

Taxman, F., & Belenko, S. (2012). *Implementing evidence-based practices in community corrections and addiction treatment*. New York, NY: Springer.

Taxman, F. S., Perdoni, M. L., & Harrison, L. D. (2007). Drug treatment services for adult offenders: The state of the state. *Journal of Substance Abuse Treatment, 32*, 239–254.

Toch, H., & Adams, K. (1986). Pathology and disruptiveness among prison inmates. *Journal of Research in Crime and Delinquency, 23*, 7–21.

Toch, H. K., Adams, K., & Grant, J. D. (1989). *Coping: Maladaption to prisons*. New Brunswick, NJ: Transaction.

Van Voorhis, P., & Presser, L. (2001). *Classification of women offenders: A national assessment of current practices*. Washington, DC: NIC.

Wexler, H. K. (2003). The promise of prison-based treatment for dually diagnosed inmates. *Journal of Substance Abuse Treatment, 25*, 223–231.

Whitten, L. (2004). *No wrong door for people with co-occurring disorders. Research News 19*. Washington, DC: National Institute on Drug Abuse, US Department of Health and Human Services.

Witt, J. C. (1986). Review of the wide range achievement test-revised. *Journal of Psychoeducational Assessment, 4*, 87–90.

Zajac, G. (2007). *Understanding and implementing correctional options that work: Offender risk and needs assessment.* [PowerPoint Slides]. Retrieved November 11, 2010, from Pennsylvania Department of Corrections Website: http://www.cor.state.pa.us/portal/server.pt/community/department_of_corrections

Ziedonis, D. M., & D'Avanzo, K. (1998). Schizophrenia and substance abuse. In H. R. Kranzler, & B. J. Rounsaville (Eds.), *Dual diagnosis and treatment: Substance abuse and comorbid medical and psychiatric disorders* (pp. 427–459). New York, NY: Marcel Dekker.

Correctional outcomes of offenders with mental disorders

Lynn A. Stewart and Geoff Wilton

Research Branch, Correctional Service Canada, 340 Laurier Ave. West, Ottawa, Ontario, Canada K0A 0P9

While there is now a considerable literature on the extent of mental disorder (MD) within correctional settings, there is much less research on the correctional outcomes of offenders with a mental disorder (OMDs). This study contributes to that knowledge base by comparing the profiles and institutional and community outcomes of federally-sentenced Canadian offenders with, and without, a MD and examines the correctional response to their management. Results showed that OMDs had higher risk and need ratings and were more likely to be serving their current sentence for a violent offense. Outcomes for OMDs were poorer as reflected by higher rates of institutional charges and transfers to segregation, and higher rates of recidivism on release. This difference holds for the recidivism analysis, even when variables related to risk are controlled. The results demonstrate the complex needs of OMDs and points to the requirement for correctional agencies to provide specialized interventions that address both their mental health and criminogenic needs. Future research is required to examine whether type of diagnosis, particularly the degree of antisocial orientation, contribute to these poorer outcomes.

Introduction

Literature review

Prevalence rates of major mental disorders (MDs) among offenders vary depending on the definition of MD adopted, the time frame applied and the population examined. Estimates range from a low of 15% (Magaletta, Diamond, Faust, Daggett, & Camp, 2009) to as high as 80% when personality and substance abuse disorders are included (Brink, 2005; Brink, Doherty, & Boer, 2001). Some of the highest rates have been found in the federal Canadian correctional system (Beaudette, Power, & Stewart, 2013; Brink et al., 2001; Motiuk & Porporino, 1991). Offenders with major mental disorders, then, can constitute a significant proportion of the offender population, posing a challenge for those mandated to provide the specialized services many require. Moreover, there is consistent evidence across constituencies that the rates of MD in offender populations have been increasing, although the reason for this is less clear (Diamond, Wang, Holzer, Thomas, & Cruser, 2001). Deinstitutionalization has been implicated in the increase (Ogloff, 2002), but at least one study failed to confirm the link between closure of psychiatric inpatient beds and increases in rates of MD in prison in the time period from the 1960s to the 1980s (Steadman, Monahan, Duffee, Hartstone, & Robbins, 1984).

While the estimates of MDs among offenders are often high, it should be noted that MDs are not rare, even in the general population. The recent national community mental health survey found that 17% of Canadians perceived themselves as being in need of mental health care within the last year (Statistics Canada, 2012). Likewise, in the US, a survey including over 20,000 adults determined that over 22% had experienced a mental health disorder in the last year, and this rate rises to 28% if a substance abuse disorder is included in the calculation (Diamond et al., 2001). Worldwide, depression is the leading cause of years lived with disability, and MD contributes more to the global burden of disease than all cancers combined (World Health Organisation, 2009).

Understanding the risk for criminal behavior posed by offenders with mental disorders is an important component in devising effective correctional supervision and intervention strategies. Over-estimating the risk can mean that individuals with these disorders are stigmatized and, as a result, the criminal justice and correctional response to their adjudication and supervision may be unjustifiably punitive or, at least, overly cautious. The consensus on the relative risk posed by individuals with MDs has evolved over the last 20 years. Despite the public's fear of individuals who are mentally ill, experts in the fields of both mental health and criminology had frequently insisted that people who are mentally ill were not more of a risk to commit acts of violence than those without a mental illness; indeed, key studies found that some kinds of serious mental illness appeared to present a protective factor, reducing the likelihood of future violence (Bonta, Law, & Hanson, 1998; Monahan et al., 2001; Quinsey, Harris, Rice, & Cormier, 2006).

Recently, however, the consensus has changed, based in part on cumulative evidence from several large scale studies (e.g. Baillargeon, Binswanger, Penn, Williams, & Murray, 2009; Vevera, Hubbard, Vesley, & Pevezova, 2005). These studies have confirmed that although the absolute amount of violent crime committed by individuals with MDs is small (most estimates are under 10%), having a diagnosis for some types of serious MD does indeed increase the risk for violence (e.g. Fazel & Grann, 2006; Walsh, Buchanan, & Fahy, 2002). A Danish study examined the mental health and correctional outcomes of 358,180 individuals drawn from a birth cohort of everyone born between 1 January 1944 and 31 December 1947. The researchers focused on the outcome for the sample of individuals who had been hospitalized because of a MD. They found that persons hospitalized for a major MD were responsible for a disproportionate percentage of violence committed by the members of the birth cohort. Men with organic psychoses and both men and women with schizophrenia were significantly more likely to be arrested for criminal violence than were persons who had never been hospitalized, even when controlling for demographic factors, substance abuse, and personality disorders (Brennan, Mednick, & Hodgins, 2000). An American study reviewing outcomes of 79,211 offenders who had received a mental diagnosis over a six year period found that those with major depressive disorder, bipolar disorders, schizophrenia, and non-schizophrenic psychotic disorders had substantially increased risks of multiple incarcerations over the six-year study period. Of these, the poorest outcomes were for inmates with bipolar disorders (Baillargeon et al., 2009).

Research also suggests that schizophrenia, or some subtypes of schizophrenia, is one of the MDs associated with criminality and particularly, with violence (e.g. Lindqvust & Allebeck, 1990; Wessely, Castle, Douglas, & Taylor, 1994). In a large scale literature review that surveyed studies that estimated the prevalence of MD in 12 countries, Fazel and Danesh (2002) found that schizophrenia was 10 times more common in prisons than would be expected based on its prevalence in the general population. An Australian study (Mullen, Burgess, Wallace, Palmer, & Ruschena, 2000) found that patients with schizophrenia were significantly more likely to be convicted for all categories of criminal offending, except sexual offenses than general population controls. Those with schizophrenia and a co-morbid substance abuse problem accounted for a disproportionate amount of offending.

Research has produced conflicting results on the role of substance abuse in increasing the risk for general criminal offending among people with MDs, but there is evidence suggesting that it plays a key role in explaining violent offending in this population. In the influential MacArthur Risk Assessment Study that examined the relationship between criminality, violence, and MDs, researchers found that substance abuse and psychopathy (particularly the criminal history aspect of psychopathy as measured by the Hare Psychopathy Checklist, rather than the emotional detachment factor) were the strongest factors contributing to risk for violence among this population (Monahan et al., 2001).

A large scale study that examined a sample of 10,059 adult residents from Epidemiologic Catchment Area study sites in the US (Eaton & Kessler, 1985), found that 8% of those with a diagnosis for schizophrenia were involved with acts of, but co-morbidity with substance abuse increased this to 30%. An earlier meta-analytic study by Bonta et al. (1998) also found that key factors contributing to risk of violent reoffending among offenders with mental disorders were antisocial personality disorder (APD), previous criminal history, and substance abuse. The authors concluded that the risk factors for criminal and violent recidivism among offenders with mental disorders are the same as for offenders without a MD; namely, factors related to the extent of the criminal history, antisocial personality, substance abuse, unemployment, and family dysfunction. Tengström, Hodgins, Grann, Långström, and Kullgren (2004) found that the key risk factor predicting violent offending was psychopathy, not general MD or substance abuse. In their sample of 78 men with a primary diagnosis of psychopathy and 202 men with a diagnosis of schizophrenia with high psychopathy scores, the non-mentally ill group diagnosed with psychopathy committed the highest numbers of offenses per year at risk.

There is a body of research investigating the role of MD in poor prison adjustment. Studies have found an association between some types of MDs and higher rates of institutional infractions (Felson, Silver, & Remster, 2008). Offenders with mental disorders with co-occurring substance abuse problems may have particularly high rates of prison misconducts (Friedmann, Melnick, Jiang, & Hamilton, 2008; Houser, Belenko, & Brennan, 2012). Researchers' debate whether it is the experience of being incarcerated that triggers mental health problems associated with prison maladjustment or whether the problems are related to pre-existing mental health problems and personality characteristics (Jiang & Fisher-Giorlando, 2002). The most consistent finding in this area reflects the results of studies examining factors related to recidivism. Namely, offenders with more antisocial traits, in particular, those with higher scores on psychopathy, are more frequently involved in misconducts and violence within correctional institutions. This appears to be true for both men and women offenders (e.g. Blackburn & Trulson, 2010; Guy, Edens, Anthony, & Douglas, 2005; Skopp, Edens, & Ruiz, 2007).

Inconclusive studies estimating the risk OMDs pose for general and violent offending may be related to the variations in the samples from which the estimates are derived, and the extent to which individuals in the samples demonstrate long term patterns of antisocial behavior. For example, there is mounting evidence that individuals with a MD fall into two main groups: the first group includes those with no history of antisocial behavior or criminality before the onset of the major mental illnesses, and the second group is comprised of 'early starters' that is, offenders with a mental disorder who display patterns of antisocial behavior from early childhood that escalate into delinquency and persistent criminality in adulthood (Hodgins, 2000; Moran & Hodgins, 2004; Mullen, 2006). Late starters whose offense histories begin after their diagnosis, can pose a risk under some conditions such as when they are under the influence of organized delusional systems with violent content, but when the negative symptoms of the illness predominate (such as social isolation and depression), they may be at lower risk for criminal and violent offending than those without a disorder (Hodgins & Janson, 2002; Hodgins, Toupin, & Côté, 1996). Individuals from this sample predominate in mental health facilities while the latter group are more common in prison settings. Studies that recruit subjects from a population of offenders are likely to find that the strength of the relationship of MD and criminal recidivism is outweighed by the impact of more robust criminal risk factors common to offender populations. The association between criminal behavior and MD within the general population, however, may be stronger since the prevalence of antisocial personality orientation and substance abuse will be much lower than in prison populations (see Bonta et al., 1998).

The current study

The Canadian federal system administers the sentences of offenders sentenced to two years or more. The current study draws from a sample of Canadian federally-sentenced OMDs and compares their outcomes to a cohort without these disorders. The study also examines the correctional response to managing these offenders by determining whether correctional staff and parole board members are less likely to grant discretionary release and more likely to impose and uphold technical violations once they were released to the community than they are for offenders without MDs.

Method

Participants

A total sample of 796 offenders (753 men and 43 women) consisting of offenders with and without a MD was obtained from two pools. One sample comprised 463 consecutive admissions to Correctional Service of Canada (CSC) at the Regional Reception and Assessment Centre (RRAC) in the Pacific region between October 2006 and December 2007. A previous study demonstrated that offenders from this sample did not differ significantly from the federal population in CSC as a whole and it was therefore concluded that the region was representative of the national population (Stewart, Wilton, & Malek, 2011). To ensure the study had enough offenders with mental health disorders for meaningful analyses, files of 333 offenders with accepted referrals to the Community Mental Health Initiative

(CMHI) were examined for potential inclusion. These offenders had been admitted to CSC within the same time period as the RRAC sample.

The total sample of 796 offenders was divided into mentally disordered and non-mentally disordered groups based on file coding that confirmed whether an offender had at least one of the following major MDs: major depression, bipolar, schizophrenia, other psychotic disorders, or anxiety disorders. The coding resulted in identifying 202 offenders from the total sample (149 from the CMHI source and 53 from the RRAC source) with a confirmed mental health diagnosis that met the criteria for this study. The remaining 594 offenders whose files had no indication that they had ever been given a mental health diagnosis included in the study comprised the comparison group. Diagnoses of personality disorders, brain injury or organic brain dysfunction, developmental disabilities or intellectual impairment, or dysthymia were not captured within the definition of major MD used for this study. Offenders with these types of diagnoses, with the exception of APD, were excluded unless they also had a diagnosis for one of the other major MDs as well. Offenders with diagnoses of APD and substance abuse disorder only do not meet criteria for inclusion in the CMHI because correctional programs, rather than mental health programs, are in place to address symptoms of these disorders. Based on previous research, we know the majority of the CSC population meet the criteria for a diagnosis with APD or substance abuse disorders (Beaudette et al., 2013; Motiuk & Porporino, 1991). As a result, both the mentally disordered group and the non-mentally disordered comparison group would have included offenders with these disorders.

Seventeen of the 43 women in the total sample were in the OMD group, constituting 8.4% of that group. The remaining 26 women were in the comparison group. Table 1 presents the breakdown by type of disorder for the 202 offenders included in the study who had a mental health diagnosis. The percentages represent the proportion of offenders who had been given a specific diagnosis; some offenders had multiple diagnoses. There were roughly equal numbers of offenders with depression, bi-polar, anxiety, and schizophrenic/psychotic disorders for men. For women, there were equal numbers of offenders with a diagnosis of depression, bi-polar, and anxiety disorders, although the low number of women offenders in the sample makes estimations of this kind uncertain. There was no difference in the proportion of disorders by gender or Aboriginal ethnicity (Aboriginal includes offenders who self-identify as being Inuit, Métis, or First Nations).

Table 1. Types of mental health disorders in the sample by gender, $n = 202$.

Type of disorder	Men $n = 185$ % (n)	Women $n = 17$ % (n)	Total $n = 202$ % (n)
Depression	26.8 (57)	31.8 (7)	27.2 (64)
Anxiety	25.8 (55)	31.8 (7)	26.4 (62)
Bipolar	23.9 (51)	31.8 (7)	24.7 (58)
Schizophrenia/schizophreniform	19.2 (41)	4.5 (1)	17.9 (42)
Other psychotic disorders	4.2 (9)	0 (0)	3.8 (9)

Note: The frequency of disorders is 235 because some offenders had more than one disorder.

Measures

Profiling information on the offenders was extracted from components of the Offender Management System (OMS), the official electronic record on all Canadian federally-sentenced offenders. This information includes demographic information as well as the results of a comprehensive assessment process conducted by specialized parole officers upon each offender's entry into the federal correctional system. It also includes sentence information, criminal history, admissions to segregation, correctional program participation, history of institutional disciplinary charges, and parole board release information.

The intake assessment process includes two principle components. The Dynamic Factors Identification and Analysis component assesses a wide variety of dynamic criminogenic risk factors grouped into seven domains: employment, marital/family, associates, substance abuse, community functioning, personal/emotional, and attitude. These factors are referred to as dynamic since they are subject to change in response to intervention. On most domains, parole officers use structured professional judgement to rate offenders on a four-point scale: (1) factor seen as an asset, (2) no current difficulty, (3) some difficulty, and (4) considerable difficulty. The substance abuse and personal emotional domains omit the factor is an asset rating, so these domains have only a three point scale. For this study, ratings of either some or considerable difficulty were considered as an indication of a need on that domain. The parole officer makes an overall need rating of 'low,' 'moderate,' or 'high' based on the results of the assessment of all domains (Brown & Motiuk, 2005).

The second component of the intake assessment involves the assessment of static risk which includes the results of an actuarial risk tool as well as a structured review of the details of the offenders' criminal histories. The Statistical Information on Recidivism-Revised (SIR-R) scale is an actuarial tool that assesses risk for general reoffending within three years of release (Nuffield, 1982). The scale is comprised of 15 static risk items such as the offender's current age, the number and type of previous offences, and pervious failures on release. Each item is weighted according to the strength of its established association with recidivism. The total score provides an overall numerical risk rating that indicates the probability of successful reintegration and places each offender in a category from very poor to very good risk. In addition to the results of the SIR-R, the parole officer also reviews a variety of static risk factors such as the volume and severity of the criminal history and the number of previous prison terms. Using structured professional judgement, parole officers provide an overall risk rating of low, moderate, or high risk based on consideration of the SIR-R results and the static risk factor analysis. CSC policy does not allow the use of the SIR-R measure for women or for Aboriginal men. Therefore, the overall risk rating for these groups is based only on the parole officers' static risk assessment. Combined, the risk and need assessment tool has a well-established association with offenders' outcome on release (Brown & Motiuk, 2005).

The Custody Rating Scale (CRS) is applied at intake to assess the appropriate security placement of offenders with determinate sentences. The CRS consists of two independently scored sub-scales: a five-item Institutional Adjustment subscale and a seven-item Security Risk subscale. Security classification is determined based on the total subscale scores, in accordance with predetermined cut-off values for allocation to minimum and maximum security (Solicitor General Canada, 1987). The final decision on the security level placement is discretionary, however, and can over-ride the CRS result.

The Computerized Assessment of Substance Abuse (CASA) evaluates the extent of substance misuse and its relationship to offending. This assessment procedure includes the results of several well-validated self-report measures of substance misuse including the 20-item Drug Abuse Screening Test (DAST; Skinner, 1982) and the Alcohol Dependency Scale (ADS; Skinner & Horn, 1984). All incoming offenders who consent to the assessment complete the ADS and DAST on a computer. The results of these measures are used to derive overall substance abuse scores and program referral recommendations.

Disciplinary charges

Minor institutional offenses are defined as any negative or non-productive inmate behavior that is contrary to institutional rules, and can include disobeying orders or being disrespectful to staff. Serious institutional offenses include breaches of security, violent or harmful acts, and repetitive violations of rules. Assaults on another inmate or staff and possession of unauthorized items are examples of serious charges. These violations are routinely recorded in OMS and were extracted for analysis for this study. To control for the period at risk, the study groups were compared on rates of charges per offender person year (OPY) incarcerated.

Transfers to segregation

There are three types of segregation transfers. Voluntary and involuntary segregation are used if the continued presence of the inmate in the general population would jeopardize the inmate's own safety, jeopardize the security of the institution, or interfere with an ongoing investigation. Disciplinary segregation is a sanction for serious disciplinary offenses. Transfers to segregation of any kind are recorded in OMS.

Parole board release decisions

The Parole Board of Canada makes parole decisions under the authority of the Corrections and Conditional Release Act. Most offenders (except those serving life sentences for murder) are eligible to apply for full parole after serving one-third of their sentence. Offenders can typically apply for day parole six months prior to their full parole eligibility dates. By law, most offenders who are serving determinate sentences and who have not been granted parole or had their parole revoked, must be released at their statutory release dates after having served two-thirds of their sentence. Statutory release does not require a decision by the Parole Board of Canada. Rarely, offenders who are assessed by the parole board as a risk to reoffend violently prior to the end of their sentence may be detained in custody until their warrants expire. For this study, information on parole board decisions was collected on each offender's first release. Differences in the proportion of offenders from both groups who were granted various forms of release were examined. In addition, for offenders on a determinate sentence (i.e. not including lifers), the proportion of the total sentence served prior to release was calculated and compared for both groups.

Correctional program assignments and completions

Within CSC, there is a menu of standardized correctional programs designed to address criminogenic needs for those at risk for reoffending. Based on the intake assessment, a correctional plan recommends participation in programs to meet the identified needs. Referrals to, and participation in, these programs are recorded centrally on the electronic database. In this study, the proportion of offenders who completed programs was compared for the two groups.

Outcomes on release

Recidivism information was collected on all offenders using Canadian Police Information Centre (CPIC) data. CPIC is the complete database recording the offense and adjudication histories on those charged by any police force in Canada. The date of the first charge following release and the date of the first charge involving a violent offense were recorded for each offender. Violent offenses were defined as homicide, manslaughter, sexual offenses, assault, and robbery. Inter-rater reliability of CPIC analysis indicated strong agreement between raters (*kappa* = .97). CPIC records permit examination of outcomes from the time of release allowing observation of all criminal involvement including the period after the federal sentence has expired. In addition, CSC maintains a database on the outcomes of offenders while under supervision. Offenders' release may be revoked and they can be returned to custody for technical reasons which can involve a degree of discretion on the part of decision-makers. Examples of technical violations are failure to attend a supervision meeting or a positive urinalysis. On the other hand, offenders will be automatically revoked and returned to custody if they have committed a new offense. In this case, no discretion is involved. The proportion of first returns to custody including those for technical violations, for an offense, and for a violent offense on the offenders' first release were recorded and compared between groups.

Procedure

The electronic files (OMS) of offenders in the sample were reviewed to determine whether there was mental health diagnosis. A coding manual was developed to guide the process (see Stewart et al., 2011 for a copy of the manual). Coding focused on review of psychology reports, intake assessments, correctional plan progress reports, and immediate needs mental health files. Offenders with an indication that a qualified clinician (psychiatrist or registered psychologist) had conferred a diagnosis of major depression, bipolar disorder, schizophrenia, schizophreniform, other psychotic disorders, or anxiety disorders were included in the OMD group. Offenders with ambiguous diagnoses (i.e. mental health professionals did not agree on the type or presence of a disorder) were not included in the study. File review for offenders from the CMHI was completed by the researcher who developed the coding manual. For the sample of offenders admitted to RRAC, this same researcher trained a team of coders to review the files using a similar manual and procedure. Inter-rater reliability on these files indicated an agreement rate of 93% and a *kappa* of .76.

The OMD group and the group without a MD were compared with appropriate inferential statistics including chi-squared tests and *t*-tests. The phi statistic is reported as an indication of the strength of the association of the variables. OPY rates were calculated to control for time-at-risk (i.e. time incarcerated or time following release) for events including institutional charges, admissions to segregation, and revocations and violent reconviction outcomes following release. For example, the total number of serious institutional charges in a group would be divided by the cumulative total time in years that the group was incarcerated – the time during which the institutional charges may have occurred.

Survival analyses, specifically, proportional hazards regression analyses, were conducted to determine the relative contribution of MD and other variables to time to first reconviction after release. Follow-up time was defined as the number of days between release and the failure event, or, for the offenders who did not fail, the days between release and date of data collection. In rare cases, the follow-up ended with the death or deportation of the offender. As with other forms of regression, survival analysis is susceptible to multicollinearity. Since failures on release were quite rare, the covariates or predictor variables selected were restricted to study group, age, DAST (drug abuse), ADS (alcohol dependence), overall criminogenic need rating, overall criminal history risk rating, rating on the criminal attitudes domain, and rating on the criminal associates domain.[1]

Results

Comparison of offender profiles

Demographic profiles of offenders with mental disorders and the cohort of offenders without MDs are presented in Table 2. There were disproportionately more White and Aboriginal offenders in the group with MDs and fewer offenders of other racial backgrounds. OMDs were less likely to be married or living common-law. Proportionately more were serving a current offense for a crime involving violence.

The average age at admission of the two groups was 35 years. The average sentence between the two groups did not differ with each group serving a mean sentence length of approximately 3.5 years.

As shown in Table 3, the overall criminogenic needs rating was significantly higher for the OMD group ($\chi^2(2) = 32.6$, $\varphi = .20$, $p < .001$). One expects the needs ratings for offenders with diagnoses of serious mental illness to be higher on factors related to their psychological functioning than for offenders without diagnoses, and this was in fact the pattern with higher ratings on the personal/emotional domain for the OMD group. However, the need ratings related to the criminal associates and attitudes domains were lower for the OMD group. These are two of the need areas most commonly cited among the 'Big Four' dynamic risk factors that contribute to criminality (Andrews & Bonta, 2010). The overall criminal risk ratings indicated that the OMD group was significantly higher risk than the comparison group ($\chi^2(2) = 17.3$, $\varphi = .15$, $p < .001$). The results of the actuarial risk assessment tool, the SIR-R, confirmed the higher risk ratings for offenders with mental disorders ($\chi^2(2) = 11.6$, $\varphi = .14$, $p = .02$).

Table 2.   Demographic and criminal profile of offenders with and without a mental disorder.

Profile variable	OMD (n = 202) % (n)	Comparison (n = 594) % (n)	χ^2	φ
Ethnicity			17.39***	.15
White	74.3 (150)	67.5 (401)		
Aboriginal	20.3 (41)	14.8 (82)		
Black	1.0 (2)	5.6 (33)		
Other	4.5 (9)	10.1 (60)		
Marital status			19.10***	.16
Married or common law	27.2 (55)	43.9 (260)		
Divorced, separated, widowed	13.4 (27)	11.3 (67)		
Single	58.9 (119)	43.6 (259)		
Unknown	.5 (1)	1.2 (7)		
Major admitting offense			57.26***	.27
Homicide or manslaughter	5.6 (12)	7.7 (46)		
Robbery	35.6 (72)	20.7 (123)		
Assault	14.4 (29)	7.1 (42)		
Sexual offenses	10.9 (22)	7.7 (46)		
Other violent offenses	7.9 (16)	6.7 (40)		
Drug offenses	2.0 (4)	18.2 (108)		
Other non-violent offenses	23.3 (47)	31.8 (189)		
Indeterminate sentences	2.0 (4)	2.2 (13)		

***$p < .001$.

The emerging literature on the impact of substance abuse on the quality of life of individuals with a MD and on their criminality required a closer look at the extent of substance abuse among these offenders. As shown in Table 3, the results on the substance abuse domain need rating as well as the self-report measures that comprise the CASA indicate that the OMD group had significantly higher rates of alcohol and drug abuse. Over 22% of OMDs had moderate or higher ratings of alcohol dependence as measured by the ADS, more than double the rate of offenders in the comparison group ($\chi^2(2) = 33.8$, $\varphi = .22$, $p < .001$) . The differences between groups were not so large for drug abuse; both groups had substantial drug abuse problems.

Correctional response

Security placement

Table 4 indicates that despite there being no differences between groups on the results of the initial CRS score ($\chi^2(2) = 2.0$, $\varphi = .05$, $p = .34$), offenders with mental disorders were significantly more likely to be placed in a maximum security institution, and less likely to be placed in a minimum security institution, than the comparison group ($\chi^2(2) = 11.2$, $\varphi = .12$, $p = .004$). The Custody Rating Score was more likely to be over-ridden to a higher level of custody for the OMD group.

Release decisions

For offenders with determinate sentences, the mean proportion of the sentence served incarcerated significantly differed between the two groups (t (696) = 4.7,

Table 3. Risk and need profiles of offenders by group.

Risk/need	OMD ($n = 200$) % (n)	Comparison ($n = 590$) % (n)	φ
Criminogenic need level			.20**
Low	6.0 (12)	19.7 (116)	
Medium	26.5 (53)	33.9 (200)	
High	67.5 (135)	46.4 (274)	
Criminal static risk level			.15**
Low	11.0 (22)	24.9 (147)	
Medium	45.5 (91)	39.2 (231)	
High	43.5 (87)	35.9 (212)	
Domain need rating			
Employment	59.0 (118)	62.5 (367)	.01
Personal/emotional	97.0 (194)	86.7 (508)	.15***
Attitude	56.0 (112)	75.6 (443)	.19***
Associates	54.5 (109)	78.8 (462)	.24***
Family/marital	53.0 (106)	45.0 (263)	.07*
Community function	46.0 (92)	45.9 (269)	.01
CASA (Substance abuse scale)	$n = 166$	$n = 549$	
ADS			.22**
None	38.6 (64)	58.8 (323)	
Low	39.2 (65)	31.9 (175)	
Moderate	10.2 (17)	5.3 (29)	
Substantial	5.4 (9)	2.7 (15)	
Severe	6.6 (11)	1.3 (7)	
DAST			.16*
None	22.9 (38)	30.6 (168)	
Low	16.3 (27)	23.0 (126)	
Moderate	28.3 (47)	16.2 (89)	
Substantial	18.1 (30)	20.8 (114)	
Severe	14.5 (24)	9.5 (52)	

*$p < .05$.
**$p < .01$.
***$p < .001$.

$p < .001$, Cohen's $d = .43$). Table 4 shows that OMDs tended to serve over half of their sentences incarcerated ($M = .55$, $SD = .18$, range $= .06–.99$), while offenders in the comparison group were incarcerated for less than half of their sentence ($M = .46$, $SD = .22$, range $= .03–1$). Of the offenders released during the period of the study, those in the OMD group were more likely to be released at their statutory release dates; in addition, proportionately fewer were granted discretionary release than the comparison group (29.4% vs. 44.8%).

Offender outcomes

Completion of program assignments

The proportion of offenders in each group who had completed one or more correctional programs while they were in prison or in the community under supervision was examined. The majority (61%) of the OMD group had completed at least one correctional program. This proportion was significantly less than the 69% of the comparison group ($\chi^2(1) = 3.9$, $\varphi = .07$, $p = .05$). The difference was due to the lower proportion of OMDs completing programs while in the community.

Table 4. Correctional response to the management of OMDs: security placement and release decisions.

Security classification	OMD % (n)	Comparison % (n)	φ
Offenders' security level			.12[**]
Minimum	18.7 (37)	29.3 (171)	
Medium	69.7 (138)	63.9 (373)	
Maximum	11.6 (23)	6.9 (40)	
Custody rating scale (CRS)			.05
Minimum	27.2 (47)	32.1 (179)	
Medium	55.5 (96)	53.8 (300)	
Maximum	17.3 (30)	14.2 (79)	
Type of release			
Day parole	29.4 (52)	44.8 (236)	.14[***]
Full parole	3.4 (6)	4.6 (24)	.03
Statutory release	61.6 (109)	46.7 (246)	.13[***]
Warrant expiry	4.0 (7)	1.9 (10)	.06
Other[a]	1.7 (3)	2.1 (11)	.01

[a]Includes deceased, court order other jurisdiction, court order freedom, and long term supervision.
[**]$p < .01$.
[***]$p < .001$.

Offenders with a mental disorder completed programs as consistently as offenders without a MD while they were incarcerated.

Institutional behavior

The correctional outcomes of offenders while incarcerated were examined by comparing the relative rates of their involvement in minor and serious institutional charges, and admissions to, and time spent in, segregation. The rate of serious institutional charges per year incarcerated was significantly greater for the OMD than the comparison group (rate ratio^2 = 1.57, 95% CI [1.32, 1.88]). Likewise, the rate of minor institutional charges was significantly greater for the OMD group (1.21; rate ratio = 1.30, 95% CI [1.16, 1.45]). The rate of voluntary and involuntary segregation admissions was also significantly greater for the OMD group (rate ratio = 1.67, 95% CI [1.14, 2.44] and 1.37, 95% CI [1.10, 1.69], respectively). The mean proportion of the time spent in segregation during the period of incarceration followed a similar pattern. The OMD group ($M = .04$, $SD = .10$) spent a significantly greater proportion of their sentences in involuntary segregation than the comparison group ($M = .02$, $SD = .06$, $t(702)$ = 2.91, $p = .004$, Cohen's $d = .22$).

Community outcomes

A survival analysis was run to test whether the survival times to first reconviction differed between OMD and comparison groups. Subsequent survival analyses included criminal risk rating, criminogenic need ratings, age at admission, and criminal attitudes and associates domain ratings as covariates to determine whether any potential differences between the two groups persist when these factors are controlled. Survival analysis also controls for the longer average follow-up time for the OMD group ($M = 854$ days, $SD = 834$) than the comparison group ($M = 760$ days, $SD = 895$, $t (702) = 4.08$, $p < .001$, Cohen's $d = .33$).

Prior to entering any covariates, the survival functions of the OMD and comparison groups differed significantly, with the OMD group being more likely to be reconvicted ($\chi^2(1) = 6.56$, $p = .01$). This result is displayed in Figure 1. The hazard ratio indicated that OMDs were 1.5 times more likely to fail than offenders without a MD.

A number of variables theoretically related to recidivism were examined in a proportional hazards regression analysis. These variables included: age at admission, DAST rating (drug abuse), ADS rating (alcohol dependence), overall criminogenic need rating, attitude domain rating, associates domain rating, and criminal history risk rating. The full model, displayed in Table 5, was significant ($\chi^2(3) = 39.30$, $p < .001$), indicating that the model predicts recidivism. The hazard ratio for the MD variable indicates that the OMD group was 1.59 times more likely to be reconvicted than the comparison group even when the other key risk variables in the model are statistically controlled.

A more parsimonious survival model was developed by running a series of hierarchical survival analyses predicting time to reconviction. Covariates other than MD were added to the model one-by-one starting with the variable supplying the greatest independent contribution to prediction. These covariates in the order that they were entered included: DAST rating (drug abuse), criminogenic need rating, attitude domain rating, age at admission, associates domain rating, and criminal risk rating. The ADS score was also considered for entry into the model but did not significantly predict survival time on its own so was dropped from the list of covariates. If a covariate was not a significant predictor of time to reconviction, it

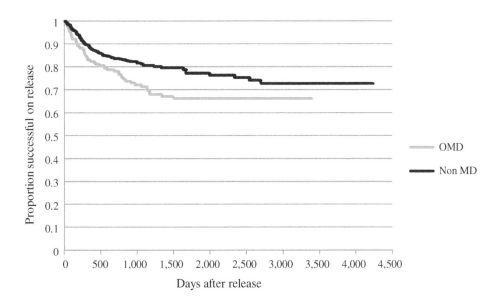

Figure 1. Survival analysis to first reconviction after release by group ($N = 704$).

Table 5. Full model predicting survival to first reconviction after release ($N = 588$).

Covariate	Wald χ^2	p	Hazard ratio
MD	5.26	.02	1.59
DAST level	14.59	<.001	1.31
Criminogenic need rating	.33	.56	1.11
Attitude domain rating	6.39	.01	1.38
Age at admission	4.43	.04	.98
Associates domain rating	.18	.67	.95
Criminal history risk rating	.97	.32	1.14
ADS level	1.05	.31	.90

was removed from the equation to reach the most parsimonious prediction model. When the attitude rating was added, criminogenic need rating was no longer a significant predictor and was removed from the model. The remaining potential covariates did not significantly add to the prediction model. The MD covariate was then added to this model. The final model, presented in Table 6, including MD, DAST rating, and attitude domain rating, significantly predicted survival to first reconviction of any type ($\chi^2(3) = 38.89$, $p < .001$). MD remained significant when drug abuse and attitude rating were controlled. After controlling for level of drug abuse (DAST) and criminogenic attitude rating, overall criminogenic need, age at admission, associates domain rating, criminal risk rating, and degree of alcohol dependence (ADS group), offenders with a MD were still over 1.5 times more likely to be reconvicted after release than the comparison group.

Another analysis was completed to assess whether the rate of revocation for technical (non-offending) reasons differed for offenders with a MD to those without a disorder. Thirty-six percent of the OMD group and 30% of the comparison group had revocations without an offense. This was a significant difference. OMDs were revoked without an offense at a rate of .38 per OPY while the comparative rate for offenders in the non-mentally disordered group was .23 per OPY (rate ratio = 1.65, 95% CI [1.22, 2.22]). The disparity could suggest the parole officers have a lesser tolerance for parole violations for offenders with mental disorders.

The rate of reconviction for a violent offense including homicide, assault, robbery, and sexual offenses as recorded on the CPIC files was very low for both groups. The rate of violent reoffending for the OMD group was 2.27 per 100 OPY; the for the comparison group it was 1.39 per 100 OPY. These rates were not significantly different (rate ratio = 1.64, 95% CI [.85, 3.07]).

Based on literature suggesting that some mental diagnoses are more often associated with antisocial or violent behavior than others, we examined the relative contribution of type of diagnosis to offenders' outcome. A survival analysis was

Table 6. Most parsimonious model predicting survival to first reconviction after release ($N = 632$).

Covariate	Wald χ^2	p	Hazard ratio
MD	6.03	.01	1.57
DAST level	22.22	<.001	1.35
Attitude rating	10.22	.001	1.40

run to test for differences among offenders with depression, anxiety, bipolar, schizophrenia, other psychotic disorders, and co-morbid disorders on time to conviction of any charge. The mean follow-up time was 2.75 years. Groups based on these types of disorders did not differ significantly in their survival functions ($\chi^2(4) = 2.84$, $p = .59$), but the number of offenders in each diagnostic category was too small to reliably detect an effect. Further research would be required to determine the relative contribution of type of MD to outcome.

Discussion

The current study examined the profile and correctional outcomes of a group of federal Canadian offenders diagnosed with a major MD relative to that of a cohort that had no mental diagnoses. An earlier study of federal offenders in Canada had concluded that offenders with serious MDs had better outcomes after a 24 month follow-up than their comparison group of offenders without a MD (Porporino & Motiuk, 1995). Despite this, the authors noted that correctional response to their institutional supervision and management on release appeared to have been more cautious as demonstrated by a lower percentage of offenders with mental disorders being granted discretionary release and a greater percentage being revoked on release for violations not related to reoffending.

The results from this current research provided a different result with respect to the outcomes of offenders with mental disorders. Firstly, the profile of offenders with mental disorders differed from the comparison group in that their criminal history risk and criminogenic needs ratings were higher. Notably, the rates of substance abuse, both for drugs and alcohol, were significantly higher for the OMD group. Offenders with mental disorders were more likely to be serving a current sentence for violence and they were significantly less likely to be married or living common-law. Despite their psychological problems, the OMD group had completed at least one correctional program while incarcerated at a rate equal to that of offenders in the comparison group. This suggests that within the structure provided by the prison setting, they are able to attend and complete programs designed to address their criminogenic needs.

Offenders with a mental disorder had poorer correctional outcomes than the comparison group. They were more likely to return to custody on technical violations and they were more likely to be reconvicted on release even when criminal history risk and criminogenic need rating, age, and substance abuse were controlled. The factors that best explained outcome on release were MD, drug abuse, and criminal attitudes.

Why were the results of the previous study by Porporino and Motiuk (1995) on mentally disordered offenders within the Canadian federal system not replicated? One explanation is that the subsample of seriously mentally ill offenders selected by Porporino and Motiuk may have had a greater representation of the type of offenders with mental disorders whose criminal careers began only with the onset of their illness. For these offenders, stabilizing their mental health problems would have reduced their risk for future reoffending. The offenders from the current study, on the other hand, may be disproportionately from the group described as early onset offenders (Hodgins, 2000). These offenders typically have long histories of antisocial behavior and persistent criminality starting in adolescence. The higher risk and need profile of the OMD group in our study would lend some support for this explanation. It is also possible that the offenders in the MD group in the current study who were identified through file review had a diagnosis on file because they had been assessed by mental health professionals after coming to the attention of prison staff because of problematic behavior. In the Porporino and Motiuk (1995) study, offenders were randomly selected and diagnosed with a MD by means of a clinical interview tool.

The correctional response to the supervision of offenders with mental disorders indicated that they were more likely to be placed in maximum security facility and less likely to be placed in a minimum security institution despite having CRS results that did not differ from the comparison group. Proportionately, fewer were granted a discretionary release and they served a greater proportion of their sentences incarcerated than the non-mentally disordered group. On release, they were more likely to be revoked for technical violations. These differences, however, cannot necessarily be ascribed to a differential correctional response due to their diagnoses. Their higher risk and need ratings and more problematic behavior while incarcerated may account for a more cautious approach to case management, rather than a concern for their mental health diagnosis.

The results have implications for correctional policy and procedures. Not surprisingly, we confirmed that offenders with a mental disorder have complex needs. They have multiple criminogenic needs that should be addressed in correctional programs in addition to mental health needs that require the provision of specialized mental health services. Stabilizing mental health is a major objective for these offenders, but interventions to address criminal risk factors must also be a key component of a comprehensive intervention strategy focused on public safety goals. It is encouraging, therefore, to note that, the offenders with mental disorders were as likely to complete a correctional program offered in the institutions as offenders without disorders. Offenders within prisons in the Canadian federal system benefit from participation in structured, well-designed correctional programs; once released in the community while they are still under warrant they continue to be provided with mental health services and supervision. An unresolved challenge to both correctional and community agencies, however, is how to bridge the period when support and supervision are provided by the criminal justice system and the time after their sentence expires when they will no longer have access to these services and support.

While the study contributes to the picture of the behavior of offenders with mental disorders while under the jurisdiction of a criminal justice agency, a number of limitations of the study must be acknowledged. This study used a convenience sample of offenders who had received a diagnosis from a qualified clinician. While the coding of files to determine the presence of a diagnosis had a high inter-rater reliability among researchers involved in the study, the reliability of rendering a diagnosis across mental health professionals is not well established. Future research could benefit from using a standardized clinical diagnostic tool to assess all offenders for the presence of a MD at intake instead of relying on file review. This would also control for another potential problem with the current design in that it required that offenders had previously gained access to mental health services, which could have been due to problematic behavior. It should also be noted that many individuals with a mental health diagnosis function well, whether as a result of treatment or spontaneous remission. A diagnosis of a MD alone does not reflect the level of impairment. This would require a measure of global functioning such as the one provided in DSM Axis V. It is even possible that the extent of the impairment due to the MD is more important to correctional outcomes than the diagnosis itself. The results also raise questions on what factors associated with having a MD account for poorer outcomes. Importantly, the study did not examine the extent to which symptoms of APD may have contributed to higher rates of involvement in institutional charges or failure on release. A closer examination of the contribution of co-occurring substance abuse problems to would also help to clarify the unique contribution of MD to criminal recidivism.

Conclusions

The current study found that offenders with mental disorders had poorer institutional and community outcomes than non-mentally disordered offenders, even when other factors related to criminality were controlled. The results demonstrate the complex needs of OMDs and the requirement for correctional agencies to be prepared to provide specialized interventions that address both their mental health and criminogenic needs.

Disclaimer

The points of view expressed in this research are those of the authors and do not necessarily reflect the views or policies of the Correctional Service of Canada.

Acknowledgments

We wish to thank the Research Branch at the Correctional Service of Canada (CSC) for their support in facilitating this project. In particular, we would like to acknowledge the contribution of Colette Cousineau and Brian Grant.

Notes

1. A larger sample would have permitted examination of a greater number of covariates, including interaction terms.
2. Rate ratios are calculated by dividing the OPY rate of one group by the other group. A rate ratio of 1 would indicate the rates of the two groups were the same. Since the 95% confidence interval excludes 1, the rate of the OMD group is significantly greater than the comparison group.

References

Andrews, D. A., & Bonta, J. (2010). *The psychology of criminal conduct* (5th ed.). Cincinnati, OH: Anderson.

Baillargeon, J., Binswanger, I. A., Penn, J. V., Williams, B. A., & Murray, O. J. (2009). Psychiatric disorders and repeat incarcerations: The revolving prison door. *American Journal of Psychiatry, 166*, 103–109.

Beaudette, J., Power, J., & Stewart, L. A. (2013). *Prevalence of mental health disorders among incoming federal offenders: Atlantic, Ontario, and Pacific regions* (Research report). Ottawa: Correctional Service of Canada.

Blackburn, A. G., & Trulson, C. R. (2010). Sugar and spice and everything nice? Exploring institutional misconduct among serious and violent female delinquents. *Journal of Criminal Justice, 38*, 1132–1140.

Bonta, J., Law, M., & Hanson, K. (1998). The prediction of criminal and violent recidivism among mentally disordered offenders: A meta-analysis. *Psychological Bulletin, 123*, 123–142.

Brennan, P. A., Mednick, S. A., & Hodgins, S. (2000). Major mental disorders and criminal violence in a Danish birth cohort. *Archives of General Psychiatry, 57*, 494–500.

Brink, J. (2005). Epidemiology of mental illness in a correctional system. *Current Opinion in Psychiatry, 18*, 536–541.

Brink, J. H., Doherty, D., & Boer, A. (2001). Mental disorder in federal offenders: A Canadian prevalence study. *International Journal of Law and Psychiatry, 24*, 339–356.

Brown, S. L., & Motiuk, L. L. (2005). *The dynamic factors identification and analysis (DFIA) component of the offender intake assessment (OIA) process. A meta-analytic, psychometric and consultative review* Research report R-164. Ottawa: Correctional Service of Canada.

Diamond, P. M., Wang, E. W., Holzer, C. E., Thomas, C. R., & Cruser, D. A. (2001). The prevalence of mental illness in prison: Review and policy implications. *Administration and Policy in Mental Health, 29*, 21–40.

Eaton, W., & Kessler, L. (1985). *The NIMH epidemiologic catchment area study. Epidemiological field methods in psychiatry.* New York, NY: Academic Press.

Fazel, S., & Danesh, J. (2002). Serious mental disorder in 23 000 prisoners: A systematic review of 62 surveys. *The Lancet, 359*, 545–550.

Fazel, S., & Grann, M. (2006). The population impact of severe mental illness on violent crime. *American Journal of Psychiatry, 163*, 1397–1403.

Felson, R. B., Silver, E., & Remster, B. (2008). Mental disorder and offending in prison. *Criminal Justice and Behavior, 39*, 125–143.

Friedmann, P. D., Melnick, G., Jiang, L., & Hamilton, Z. (2008). Violent and disruptive behavior among drug-involved prisoners: Relationship with psychiatric symptoms. *Behavioral Sciences & the Law, 26*, 389–401.

Guy, L. S., Edens, J. F., Anthony, C., & Douglas, K. S. (2005). Does psychopathy predict institutional misconduct among adults? A meta-analytic investigation. *Journal of Consulting and Clinical Psychology, 73*, 1056–1064.

Hodgins, S. (2000). The etiology and development of offending among persons with major mental disorders: Conceptual and methodological issues and some preliminary findings. In S. Hodgins (Ed.), *Violence among the mentally III* (pp. 89–160). Dordrecht: Kluwer Academic.

Hodgins, S., & Janson, C. (2002). *Criminality and violence among the mentally disordered.* New York, NY: Cambridge University Press.

Hodgins, S., Toupin, J., & Côté, G. (1996). Schizophrenia and antisocial personality disorder: A criminal combination. In L. B. Schlesinger (Ed.), *Explorations in criminal psychopathology: Clinical syndromes with forensic implications* (pp. 217–237). Springfield, IL: Charles C. Thomas.

Houser, K. A., Belenko, S., & Brennan, P. K. (2012). The effects of mental health and substance abuse disorders on institutional misconduct among female inmates. *Justice Quarterly, 29*, 799–828.

Jiang, S., & Fisher-Giorlando, M. (2002). Inmate misconduct: A test of the deprivation, importation, and situational models. *The Prison Journal, 82*, 335–358.

Lindqvist, P., & Allebeck, P. (1990). Schizophrenia and crime. A longitudinal follow-up of 644 schizophrenics in Stockholm. *The British Journal of Psychiatry, 157*, 345–350.

Magaletta, P. R., Diamond, P. M., Faust, E., Daggett, D. M., & Camp, S. D. (2009). Estimating the mental illness component of service need in corrections: Results from the Mental Health Prevalence Project. *Criminal Justice and Behavior, 36*, 229–244.

Monahan, J., Steadman, H., Silver, E., Appelbaum, P., Robbins, P., Mulvey, E., ... Banks, S. (2001). *Rethinking risk assessment: The MacArthur study of mental disorder and violence.* New York, NY: Oxford University Press.

Moran, P., & Hodgins, S. (2004). The correlates of comorbid antisocial personality disorder in schizophrenia. *Schizophrenia Bulletin, 30*, 791–802.

Motiuk, L. L., & Porporino, F. J. (1991). *The prevalence, nature and severity of mental health problems among federal male inmates in Canadian penitentiaries.* (Research Report R-24). Ottawa: Research Branch, Correctional Service of Canada.

Mullen, P. E. (2006). Schizophrenia and violence: From correlations to preventive strategies. *Advances in Psychiatric Treatment, 12*, 239–248.

Mullen, P. E., Burgess, P., Wallace, C., Palmer, S., & Ruschena, D. (2000). Community care and criminal offending in schizophrenia. *The Lancet, 355*, 614–617.

Nuffield, J. (1982). *Parole decision making in Canada: Research towards decisions guidelines.* Ottawa: Department of the Solicitor General Canada.

Ogloff, J. R. P. (2002). Identifying and accommodating the needs of mentally ill people in gaols and prisons. *Psychiatry, Psychology and Law, 9*(1), 1–33.

Porporino, F. J., & Motiuk, L. L. (1995). The prison careers of mentally disordered offenders. *International Journal of Law and Psychiatry, 18*, 29–44.

Quinsey, V. L., Harris, G. T., Rice, M. E., & Cormier, C. A. (2006). *Violent offenders: Appraising and managing risk* (2nd ed.). Washington, DC: American Psychological Association.

Skinner, H. A. (1982). The drug abuse screening test. *Addictive Behaviors, 7*, 363–371.

Skinner, H. A., & Horn, J. L. (1984). *Alcohol dependence scale (ADS): User's guide.* Toronto: Addiction Research Foundation.

Skopp, N. A., Edens, J. F., & Ruiz, M. A. (2007). Risk factors for institutional misconduct among incarcerated women: An examination of the criterion-related validity of the Personality Assessment Inventory. *Journal of Personality Assessment, 88*, 106–117.

Solicitor General Canada. (1987). *Development of a security classification model for Canadian federal offenders.* Ottawa: Correctional Service of Canada.

Statistics Canada. (2012). Canadian community health survey: Mental health 2012. Retrieved from: http://www.statcan.gc.ca/daily-quotidien/130918/dq130918a-eng.htm

Steadman, H. J., Monahan, J., Duffee, B., Hartstone, E., & Robbins, P. C. (1984). The impact of state mental hospital deinstitutionalization on United States prison populations, 1968–1978. *Journal of Criminal Law & Criminology, 75*, 474–490.

Stewart, L.A. Wilton, G., & Malek, A. (2011). *Validation of the computerised mental health screening system (CoMHISS) in a federal male offender population.* Ottawa: Correctional Service of Canada.

Tengström, A., Hodgins, S., Grann, M., Långström, N., & Kullgren, G. (2004). Schizophrenia and criminal offending: The role of psychopathy and substance use disorders. *Criminal Justice and Behavior, 31*, 367–391.

Vevera, J., Hubbard, A., Vesely, A., & Papezova, H. (2005). Violent behaviour in schizophrenia: Retrospective study of four independent samples from Prague, 1949 to 2000. *British Journal of Psychiatry, 187*, 426–430.

Walsh, E., Buchanan, A., & Fahy, T. (2002). Violence and schizophrenia: Examining the evidence. *The British Journal of Psychiatry, 180*, 490–495.

Wessely, S. C., Castle, D., Douglas, A. J., & Taylor, P. J. (1994). The criminal careers of incident cases of schizophrenia. *Psychological Medicine, 24*, 483–502.

World Health Organisation. (2009). Global health risks: Mortality and burden of disease attributable to selected major risks. Retrieved from http://www.who.int/healthinfo/global_burden_disease/GlobalHealthRisks_report_full.pdf

Service utilization in a cohort of criminal justice-involved men: implications for case management and justice systems

Roberto Hugh Potter

Department of Criminal Justice, College of Health and Public Affairs, University of Central Florida, PO Box 161600, Orlando, FL 32816, USA

In the era of re-entry, a great deal of attention has been paid to the 'risk-need-responsivity' model. Most attention to the utilization of services designed to meet need has focused on post-release behaviors. However, little attention has been paid to the pre-incarceration utilization of services that might influence receptivity to post-release utilization. Using constructs borrowed from health services utilization, the current paper examines the associations among CJ-involvement, social and health services utilization, and health status in a cohort of CJ-involved men living in the community. Results from the current cohort, combined with those of previous research, suggest that follow-through on services by released individuals' remains problematic. Suggestions for future research and questions about the role of criminal justice agencies in improving follow-through are raised.

Problem statement

Issues of linkage to services for returning prisoners and inmates have been in the forefront of re-entry programming for more than a decade now. With the development of the 'risk-need-responsivity' (RNR) model (Andrews & Bonta, 2010; Lowenkamp & Latessa, 2005), it has become important to identify the types of services needed, rather than just throwing services at re-entering individual. In the narrower discussion of inmate/prisoner re-entry (from incarceration to the community) the focus is generally on criminogenic risk reduction. Within those criminogenic needs are a range of social service needs that, while perhaps not in themselves criminogenic (Andrews & Bonta, 2010), support the reduction of criminogenic risk. These social services include housing, job preparation and placement, education/training, and so forth. Physical health and behavioral health services may also play a role in the lives of returning persons, as many health conditions are found in disproportionate levels among jail and prison populations. In a broader discussion of re-entry, whether social/health services dominate the conversation is an open question.

This paper examines the associations among CJ-involvement, social and health services utilization, and health status in a cohort of CJ-involved men living in the community. It also examines research on utilization of such services by CJ-involved persons. The results will, hopefully, inform the refinement of the roles of criminal justice agencies, social service, public health, and healthcare delivery organizations in the development of community-based systems of care to reduce criminal justice involvement, improve public safety, and reduce health and social disparities.

Exactly where and when one's criminal justice involvement begins and ends ranges from brief to life-long, continuous and discontinuous, in custody and/or under supervision, making it difficult to state one's 'criminal status' as something akin to a chronic disease. While most people under the supervision of correctional agencies are in the community on any given day – on pre-trial release, probation, or parole – many more criminal justice-involved (CJ-involved) persons are released without supervision at various points in the process. In a sense, everyone 'booked' into a jail and released back into the community is a 'returning' inmate – only the length of detention varies. And, once released without supervision, does the CJ-involvement truly end?

For the purposes of correctional health coverage, the Supreme Court of the United States has determined that the criminal justice system is responsible for health care from the point at which a police pursuit begins until the individual is released from a correctional facility (Anno, 2001). But, when an individual is released from incarceration (especially local and state), the mandate to provide health care vanishes.

The question of how CJ-involved persons utilize community resources prior to and following detention events appears to be relatively unexamined. Further, how utilization of community resources, including physical and behavioral health services, is related to criminal behavior pre- and post- CJ-involvement is another area where relatively little empirical knowledge seems to exist. It might be argued that physical health services, as well as behavioral (mental health and substance use treatment) health services, are among those non-criminogenic needs to be addressed for CJ-involved persons, regardless of the length of time they spend in detention/incarceration or their supervision status at the time of release.

A distinction between 'availability', 'access', and 'utilization' of services may be necessary. In some instances, individuals do not utilize services because those services are not available in a specific community. Access to services becomes a somewhat more complicated item. Gulliford and colleagues (2002) separate access to healthcare into four categories, which we believe can be expanded to services for CJ-involved persons:

> If services are available and there is an adequate supply of services, then the opportunity to obtain health care exists, and a population may 'have access' to services. The extent to which a population 'gains access' also depends on financial, organisational (*sic*) and social or cultural barriers that limit the utilisation (*sic*) of services. Thus access measured in terms of utilisation (*sic*) is dependent on the affordability, physical accessibility and acceptability of services and not merely adequacy of supply. Services available must be relevant and effective if the population is to 'gain access to satisfactory health outcomes'. The availability of services, and barriers to access, have to be considered in the context of the differing perspectives, health needs and material and cultural settings of diverse groups in society. Equity of access may be measured in terms of the availability, utilisation or outcomes of services. Both horizontal and vertical dimensions of equity require consideration.

In short, availability affects access which affects the actual use of available services, and all of these affect outcomes. Just building the opportunity does not mean the service will be used. Quality and acceptability of services are also factored into the utilization equation. The utilization of services may not determine outcomes. In RNR model, this would be the responsivity component.

In the next section, we will explore the limited literature on social and health service utilization among CJ-involved persons. How mechanisms such as judicial and probation/parole conditions can be employed to enhance utilization of available resources will be discussed later.

Literature review

Pre-incarceration utilization of services

As noted above, relatively few studies of pre-incarceration utilization of social services are presented in the criminal justice and criminological literature. For the criminal justice literature, such studies are found primarily in the area of substance abuse treatment and post-release behavior (Simpson & Knight, 2007; Wexler & Fletcher, 2007). There is a strong focus on utilization of substance use treatment prior to incarceration, as might be expected. A second area of focus is on the prevalence of homelessness among individuals treated for substance use disorders prior to incarceration, and some lesser attention paid to sources of income. A final area of focus in some studies of pre-incarceration service utilization is education (Steurer, Smith, & Tracy, 2001).

In the public health domain, pre-incarceration utilization of social services is most often studied in relation to HIV treatment during incarceration (e.g. Chen et al., 2011). There, the attention is mostly directed toward pre-incarceration utilization of medication, housing, and other services covered by 'Ryan White' funding for persons living with HIV. 'Ryan White funds' refer to a United States federal program of support for persons living with HIV (Ryan White Comprehensive AIDS Resources Emergency Act of 1990). For those not utilizing Ryan White services, the focus is sometimes on pre-incarceration sources of income, as well as housing status.

In the end, little empirical information about the utilization of social and health-related services among those entering jails or prison is published. Among the best sources of information that do exist are the National Inmate Survey and the National Prisoner Survey from the Bureau of Justice Statistics. We will return to data from those surveys in the analysis section.

Post-release utilization of services

Results from early large-scale prison re-entry program evaluations do not offer great hope for the utilization of services once prisoners are released back into the community. Lattimore and Visher (2009), reporting on the evaluation of the Serious and Violent Offender Re-entry Initiative (SVORI) did not measure pre-incarceration utilization of social and health services, but did ask returning persons to predict the needs they would have upon release in those two domains and others. They conclude that access to services was 'greatly increased', for SVORI participants relative to comparisons, but that receipt of post-release services was lower than the need. Females in the SVORI evaluation reported higher need and receipt of services than did the men, but the drop off in service utilization was about the same for both sexes. Over time, SVORI participants' utilization of post-release services declined to match that of the control group. That is, access to services was increased, but utilization was not.

Two of the few areas where published information about prisoner health post-release can be found are in the areas of tuberculosis and HIV. Overall, the evidence that most people who obtain treatment in correctional settings for diseases as diverse as HIV and TB improve their health status while incarcerated is robust. That is, prison-based health care is effective. After release to the community, however, the picture becomes bleaker.

Springer et al. (2004), Stephenson et al. (2005), Baillargeon et al. (2009), and Wohl et al. (2011), provided evidence that individuals living with HIV tended to get healthier while incarcerated, but were either lost to follow-up in the community or returned to prison in poor health from the community. Reznick, McCartney, Gregorich, Zack, and Feaster (2013) reported similar results with adherence to HIV medications and return to jail or prison among participants in an HIV re-entry program, regardless of post-release support condition. HIV is among the few diseases for which we have had relatively strong community continuity of care systems. Thus, whether we should expect those with other diseases with fewer community resources devoted to continuity of care to demonstrate more positive results is an open question. Likewise, the impact of universal health insurance mandates on adherence and follow-through to services remains to be seen.

Individuals enter the criminal justice process with a range of deficits, as predicted by the Problem Syndrome approach (Donovan & Jessor, 1985; Jessor & Jessor, 1977) and the Epidemiological Criminology framework (Akers, Potter, & Hill, 2013). Yet, we have relatively little published documentation of those needs, how such needs are addressed while incarcerated, or how those needs are addressed upon return to the community (availability and access). The present paper examines the self-reported and clinically documented services utilized by a group of CJ-involved men in the community to determine whether any associations among health, criminal, and social service utilization exist that can inform efforts to address multiple problem areas among this group.

Methodology

Recruitment process

These data were collected as part of a demonstration project funded by the Florida Department of Health to focus on HIV testing for 'vulnerable populations', in this case men involved in the criminal justice system. Our program was a replication of an earlier utilization of the brief intervention in DeKalb County, Georgia. The target audience for the MISTERS (Men in STD Training and Empowerment Research Study) program in Orange County (Florida) was men who had been released from a minimum 48 h of detention or imprisonment in the 12 months prior to their screening. We chose 48 h because the national average between arrest and bonding out of jail (making bail) for those booked on felony charges is around 48 h (Cohen & Reaves, 2007). As it turns out, data from Orange County Corrections Department demonstrated that the average release time for the county jail was even briefer, closer to 24 h before around half of all those booked were released. The Orange MISTERS project was designed to evaluate whether a 10-h brief intervention could lower risk of contracting STDs/HIV, enhance employability, and reduce likelihood of further criminal behavior. Primary oversight of the recruitment process was provided by the lead community agency, Nehemiah Education and Economic Development, Inc. (NEED).

Data collection

Materials and methods

The data collection for the Orange MISTERS project began during June, 2009. Criminal justice-involved men were recruited by outreach workers employed by NEED in the east Orange County and Eatonville area. Advertisement of the project included posters, flyers and business cards given to potential participants by outreach workers. Outreach workers also visited probation offices, popular 'hang out' spots and labor offices within the target community in search of candidates for the MISTERS program.

Participants for the MISTERS program were screened using a set of criteria including having spent at least 48 h in jail during the past year, having had sex at least once within the past year, and not having a prior sex offense history. Those eligible were asked if they would like to participate in the MISTERS program. The provision of health screening services, on-going health care for those who met income eligibility requirements, the 10 h brief intervention, as well as the data collection component of the project was explained to the men.

Men who agreed to participate were then scheduled for a visit to Orange Blossom Family Health Center (OBFHC) where they completed the baseline questionnaire and received HIV, Chlamydia, gonorrhea, and other disease screenings if ordered by the health clinic staff. This paper explores the utilization of social and health services in the 12 months prior to program participation, outcomes of the disease testing process, and the criminal histories reported among the men. The cohort we report on here is a convenience sample of CJ-involved men who self-selected to participate, without a comparison or control group.

Participants were asked to complete a lengthy base-line questionnaire prior to receipt of the health screening services. Consistent with the consent process approved by the University of Central Florida (UCF) Institutional Review Board, men were able to refuse to complete the form and still receive services. In year one of the project we utilized the same data collection instrument as in the original Georgia study; in years two and three we used the CDC Program Evaluation Management System questionnaire. Men who were comfortable completing the form on their own did so; men who needed assistance completing the form were assisted by the outreach workers. De-identified data forms were delivered to the UCF staff for coding and analysis. The demographic and criminal justice history data are used to describe the respondents in this paper, along with self-reported criminal histories and prior social and health services utilization data.

Disease testing for participants in the project was conducted at Orange Blossom Family Health Center, a federally qualified health care center. All participants were first given a health questionnaire and then screened for HIV and three other STDs (Gonorrhea, syphilis and herpes). If indicators of an increased risk for Hepatitis C were discovered during the health screening interview, participants were also given a test for Hepatitis C. Throughout the project, 589 baseline interviews were conducted with participants, 518 (88%) of which had a linked disease testing history through Orange Blossom Family Health Center. Overall, 88% of the men initially recruited into the program received disease screening services.

Results

Demographics

All participants in the Orange MISTERS project were male. The age distribution of baseline questionnaire respondents ranged from 18 to 61 with a mean of 34 years (median = 32.5). Most respondents were African–American (78.1%) with Hispanic/Latino and white respondents making up 8.8 and 7.3% respectively. The relationship status of most respondents was single or never married (66%) with divorced (13%) and married (10%) making up the next two largest groups. Most respondents reported living with a family member or partner (68.1%), though living alone (8.5%), living in a shelter (8.1%) and living outdoors or on the street (6.8%) were also reported. Baseline demographic categories (age, race) included those which were comparable with prior HIV testing in correctional populations in Florida (MacGowan et al., 2009). With the exception of the over-representation of

Table 1. Demographic comparison of national-level corrections populations and the orange MISTERS participants.

	Jail Inmates 2002[*]	Prisoners 2004[**]	Orange MISTERS
Age	Median = 30	Median = 35	Median = 32
Race			
Black	40%	42%	79%
White	36%	47%	7%
All others	24%	11%	14%
Education	Median < high school	Median = 11 years	Median = 11 years
Marital status			
Married	16%	26%	20%
Never	60%	45%	66%
Div/sep/widowed	24%	29%	14%
Current or conviction charge type			
Violent	25%	12%	33%
Property	24%	21%	17%
Drug	25%	7%	25%
Probation violation	NA	NA	10%
Public order	25%	24%	2%
Traffic	NA	NA	11%
Probation status at arrest			
On probation	34%		41%
On parole	13%		8%
No status	47%		51%
Pre-arrest employment			
Employed	71%	71%	13%
Unemployed	29%	29%	87%
Homeless			
Past year	14%	4%	16%

[*]Maruschak (2006).
[**]Maruschak (2008).

African-Americans, the participants were similar to those surveyed in the 2002 National Inmate Survey and 2004National Prisoner Survey (see Table 1).

Criminal justice history – static factors

Although the program required at least two nights' stay in jail or prison in the 12 months prior to enrollment, the number of nights spent inside varied from one night to twenty-eight years. The mean and median number of nights spent incarcerated on the respondents' last arrest event were 471 and 57, respectively. Fifty-three percent of respondents spent 60 days or less in jail upon their last arrest, 31% spent fifteen days or less and 24% spent six days or less in jail (anything over 365 days was likely a prison sentence).

This was not a cohort of shrinking violets. Two-thirds of the respondents reported commission of at least one misdemeanor in their lifetime. Slightly more (71%) reported at least one felony offense in their lifetime. Respondents provided the reasons for their last arrest prior to program enrollment. The most commonly reported offense involved illegal substances ($n = 137$). These were followed closely by crimes of violence ($n = 120$), and an additional 35 cases of resisting arrest, and 26 weapons charges. Property-related crimes ($n = 91$) was the next most frequently reported category. Traffic offenses, especially driving without a valid license ($n = 48$) and driving under the influence ($n = 22$) were also reported, along with 11 'public order' offenses. Being arrested for violation of a probation or parole order was reported by 56 respondents. Since a respondent could report more than one offense at the arrest prior to participation, only frequencies are reported here.

All of the respondents had been incarcerated at least once, so the next question of interest is how many had been on probation at some point in their life. Among all participants in the program, 68% reported having some lifetime history of being on probation. Respondents on probation at the time of the interview (41% of total), reported probation periods ranged from 1 month to 30 years (average 35 months; median 20 months). Unfortunately, we are unable to determine whether this was a misdemeanor or felony probation, or both for life-time or present supervision.

One possible proxy for this level of supervision information among those currently on probation is the length of probation sentence. In this case, about one-third (33%) of the respondents reported 12 or fewer months of supervision, suggesting they were on county (misdemeanor) probation. The remaining two-thirds were likely on probation supervision by the state Department of Corrections for a felony conviction. Overall, those on any probation supervision reported a mean 15 months of supervision, with a range of one to 360 months (SD = 36 months).

Although Florida effectively abolished its parole system in the 1990s, 8% of the respondents reported being on parole at the time of program enrollment. It is possible those with longer reported periods of incarceration were released on parole from sentences imposed when parole was still an option. It is also possible some of the participants were paroled from other state systems and living in Florida. Lifetime parole experience was reported by about twice as many (16%) as those currently on parole.

Six percent reported currently being under both probation and parole supervision at entry into the program. Overall, 43% ($n = 253$) reported being under some form of criminal justice supervision at enrollment.

Health status

Before their initial physical examination at OBFHC, the men were asked to list the number of diseases they knew they currently had. Only five percent noted any existing disease conditions, and only (1%) reported two or more disease conditions. With the exception of one individual, all of those reporting a current disease state were African–American. When asked about their perceived general health status, 24% responded 'excellent', another 24% responded 'very good', 37% 'good', 12% 'fair', and 3% responded 'poor'. Among those reporting one existing known disease, 71% ($n = 12$) still responded their general health was at least 'good', while all (100%; $n = 6$) of those with two or more known diseases responded with at least 'good'.

Participants were asked to indicate what sorts of health problems they had suffered in the previous 12 months at the baseline interview. Of the respondents, 545 (93%) provided consistent answers to the problem categories. The most frequently reported problem involved dental issues (17%), followed by vision problems (14%), hypertension (10%), 'foot' problems (8%), stomach and mental health problems (6% each). Back and spinal problems (3%), heart problems and diabetes (2% each), along with asthma, hepatitis C, and cancer in the previous 12 months were also reported by participants at intake. Other than the dental and vision

Table 2. Health problem comparisons – national-level corrections populations and the orange MISTERS participants.

Medical problem	Jail Inmates, 2002[*]	National Total	Prisoners, 2004[**] State	Federal	Orange MISTERS[***]
Chronic diseases					
Arthritis	13%	23%	15%	12%	11%
Hypertension	11%	32%	14%	13%	10%
Asthma	10%	8%	9%	7%	<1%
Heart problems	6%	12%	6%	6%	2%
Renal (kidney) problems	4%	2%	3%	3%	<1%
Diabetes	3%	11%	4%	5%	2%
Hepatitis (unspecified)	3%	27% – A	5%	4%	<1%
		5% – B			<1%
		1% – C			<1%
Liver problems	1%	1%	1%	1%	<1%
Infectious diseases					
TB (lifetime)	4%	4%	9%	7%	NA
HIV	1%	5%	2%	1%	2%[a]
Other sexually-transmitted diseases (STDs)	1%	<1%	1%	<1%	3%[a]
Dental	NA	NA	NA		17%
Vision	NA	NA	NA		14%

[*]Maruschak (2006).
[**]Maruschak (2008). Only survey to ask about specific variants of hepatitis virus.
[***]Past 12 months.
[a]Test result.

problems recorded here, the results are similar to those observed in the national-level studies described above (see Table 2).

A core objective of the original project was to establish a 'medical home' for the participants with OBFHC. This required first a physical examination at OBFHC, provided at no cost to the men. Information provided by OBFHC staff showed a rather poor follow-through on the physical examination. Forty-four percent ($n = 260$) of the 589 men who provided a baseline interview did not show up for the physical at OBFHC. It should be noted that the OBFHC facility was located several miles from the NEED offices, and even though bus passes were provided for travel to the OBFHC facility, the distance and need for an appointment were reported to be a deterrent for many men, according to the case workers. Unfortunately, we are unable to cross-tabulate the self-reported prior year health problems with diagnoses due to the confidentiality guarantees between OBFHC and the evaluation team.

Among those who did report and receive a diagnosis, 16% (56 of 351) opted to receive only a HIV test, and no further diagnostic exams. Of the non-STD disorders, 28 men were diagnosed with 'multiple complaints', 28 with hypertension, 19 with musculoskeletal disorders, 10 with hyperlipidemia (cholesterol), nine with pulmonary disorders, seven with psychiatric disorders, and one or two cases across a range of disorders from pain to obesity and wound care.

Service utilization

Health-related services

Respondents were asked to indicate whether they had received a range of services in the 12 months prior to program enrollment. Among the health-related services listed, relatively few reported receiving such services in the prior year. Fifty-five percent reported receiving a HIV test in the 12 months prior to program enrollment. Regrettably, we did not record the location at which the test was received.

Only 12% of the respondents reported receiving other medical services of the course of the previous year. Seven percent of the respondents reported receiving mental health or STD services in the 12 months before coming to the program. Only (4%) reported receiving non-jail-based substance abuse treatment in the previous year. A slightly higher proportion (5%) reported participating in the CHOICES drug treatment program offered at the Orange County jail.

Social service utilization

Other social services related to the needs of re-entering persons were also gauged. The least frequently received service was legal assistance (3%). Housing services were utilized by only (5%) of the respondents, probably reflecting the low level of homelessness reported. Fifteen percent of the respondents reported receipt of employment services in the previous year. Just over half (50.4%) reported receiving either food stamps or some other form of food assistance in the year before program participation.

Associations

The relationships among criminal history, self-reported and clinically-determined health status, and the utilization of a range of health and social services within the

12 months prior to program enrollment can now be assessed. Because the men in this sample were released from incarceration in the previous year, we will begin with associations between supervision status, health outcomes, and service utilization.

Supervision status

As noted earlier, 41% of the men reported being on either probation or parole at the time of program enrollment. Collapsing those two variables created a variable titled supervision status, with values currently 'under supervision' or 'no supervision'. There were no statistically significant associations observed between supervision status and any of the measures of health conditions or service utilization (see Table 3 for a listing of services). A similar analysis was performed just for those on probation with the same results.

Reporting having a history of committing a felony during their lifetime does appear to have an association with receipt of food assistance X^2 (1, $N = 589$) = 13, $p < .000$, mental health X^2 (1, $N = 589$) = 5.8, $p < .01$, and general medical services X^2 (1, $N = 589$) = 7.2, $p < .01$, in the 12 months prior to program enrollment. In this case it appears that those with a felony in their pasts were more likely to report receiving these services than those without a felony. Examining the association between self-perceived health status and a past felony we find a statistically signifi-cant relationship X^2 (4, $N = 565$) = 10.9, $p < .03$. Age (measured categorically) was also significantly associated with having committed a felony at least once lifetime X^2 (3, $N = 585$) = 23, $p < .000$.

HIV testing

The most frequently reported health-related service in the previous 12 months was receipt of a test for HIV. Again the services mental health treatment X^2 (1, $N = 589$) = 7.6, $p < .01$, food assistance X^2 (1, $N = 589$) = 9.5, $p < .002$ and general medical services X^2 (1, $N = 589$) = 6.2, $p < .01$, return significant associations with this vari-able. They are joined by receipt of services at an STD clinic X^2 (1, $N = 589$) = 3.9, $p < .05$, and participation in drug treatment services outside of jail X^2 (1, $N = 589$) = 6.6, $p < .01$, as well. It appears that those who were tested for HIV were more likely to receive these services than were those without a test in the prior year.

Table 3.   Services utilized in 12 months prior to program enrollment.

Past-year service utilization	Yes (%)	No (%)
Health-related		
Medical	68(12)	521(88)
HIV test	324(55)	263(45)
STD services	40(7)	549(93)
Mental health	41(7)	548(93)
Substance abuse treatment	25(4)	546(96)
Social services		
Employment	89(15)	500(85)
Food assistance	297(51)	291(49)
Housing assistance	29(5)	560(95)
Legal services	19(3)	570(97)

Curiously, there was no association between receipt of a test for HIV in the year prior to program enrollment and actually testing positive for HIV.

Limitations

The first limitation of this study is the nature of the sample. The project targeted men in communities deemed vulnerable for HIV acquisition. The over-representation of African–Americans in the sample reflects this fact. The men were self-selected volunteers. While on many demographic variables they match up well with the two national samples of inmates and prisoners, we cannot suggest that our results should be generalized to other communities around the nation. There is also the fact that all of our participants were male, so we cannot speak to the experiences of CJ-involved women directly. Next, much of the data reported here is self-report and self-perception. Thus, without objective clinical data for health status and agency records to verify receipt of services, we cannot say definitively what services the men may have received in the 12 months prior to joining our project. Finally, because we are reporting only descriptive information here, no indications of what variables 'cause' any of the observations can be made.

Discussion

As a measure of receipt of health and social services among CJ-involved men in the community, these results suggest that such services are received infrequently. With the exception of food assistance and HIV testing, no single service was utilized by more than 15% of the men between the time they got out of detention and coming to the project. One's current supervision status seems to have no association with either health status or receipt of services. Having a history of committing a felony offense does appear to raise the probability one will utilize these services, but only marginally. The same can be observed for having received a test for HIV in the previous year. We are limited in our ability to determine whether it is something in the process of HIV testing that makes these connections. And, failing to measure where the HIV testing occurred limits our ability to say whether these tests and potential links to services are happening in a correctional facility or in the community at the offices of a non-profit agency or health department.

Akers et al. (2013) raise the hypothesis that the same risk dimension underlies both criminal and health risk behaviors. To this we would add failure to follow-through on those services designed to address criminogenic and health risk behaviors. Many CJ-involved individuals come to the system with a track record of failure to follow-through on educational, health, and social welfare activities that had been recommended for them. Given the relatively brief time most CJ-involved persons spend in direct custody, the likelihood that the criminal justice system will have much impact on prior behavioral patterns seems relatively low. It is therefore unclear from where our expectations of post-release supervision come. Unfortunately, the follow-up efforts of our community peer outreach workers to ascertain health and social service follow-through by the MISTERS clients were not terribly successful, so we are unable to determine whether our program increased such follow-through.

These data and those presented in the literature review section bring us to a discussion of the relative roles of criminal justice, public health, health care providers, and social service providers in the lives of CJ-involved persons. As the

'Affordable Care Act' comes into implementation phase, more pressure is being brought on correctional agencies, especially jails, to enroll low-income, uninsured individuals into the universal health insurance plan. Discharge planners are already becoming fixtures in prison systems and some large and medium sized jails to assist with re-entry planning and making linkages to community organizations to provide needed services.

Potter and Rosky (2012) have outlined intersections between criminal justice and public health/health care systems. Data such as those presented here and in the literature review spur us to become more specific. For example, what is the role of the criminal justice system in compelling CJ-involved persons to utilize needed services? Even compulsory receipt of treatment for infectious diseases such as tuberculosis requires judicial intervention (Bayer & Dupuis, 1995). Specialty courts such as drug, mental health, and veterans' courts operate on a combination of state coercion and rehabilitation (Birgden, 2004).

Even though being on any form of community supervision appeared to have no association with receipt of services in this cohort, the question of whether making receipt of services a requirement or condition of supervision – beyond what are normally associated with supervision – should be raised. That is, if it requires threat of sanction to ensure that persons with access to a needed service actually use that service, should we make it a condition of pre-trial release, probation or parole? Or, in keeping with studies of readiness for change and responsivity (Ward, Day, Howells, & Birgden, 2004), do we accept that some persons are simply not aware of or ready to begin changing their behaviors? Regrettably, we were unable to tap whether those participating in our program had been ordered to any form of treatment as a condition of community supervision.

Here the criminological concern with 'net-widening' (Blomberg, 1995; Frazier, Richards, & Potter, 1983) meets the 'differing perspectives, health needs and material and cultural settings of diverse groups in society' outlined by Gulliford et al. (2002). Do we wish to utilize the coercive power of the state to ensure the accomplishment of non-criminal justice outcomes, regardless of the potential positive benefit? Do we want to place members of already vulnerable social groups under even more scrutiny by the state? Are the individual and social goods achieved by coercing CJ-involved, but not necessarily under supervision, persons into utilizing services determined to meet their 'needs' worth the expansion of state power into their lives?

The expectations of follow-through by CJ-involved persons and over what period of time are more than just abstract, academic questions. Likewise, what outcomes should be produced by intervention programs and how long should those effects last need to be clarified. Are such programs supposed to operate like vaccinations in that once you complete the vaccination sequence you will have immunity for some (un)specified period of time? Or, like correctional experiences among CJ-involved persons, are the effects intermittent, discontinuous, and/or time-limited?

Summary

The published literature on CJ-involved persons' follow-through on utilization of a range of social and health-related services is not encouraging, and the results presented for the Orange MISTERS cohort continue this disappointing trend. We found that commission of at least one felony during the respondents' lifetimes and having had a HIV test in the past 12 months were associated with the utilization of health and social services since their last release from incarceration. Unfortunately, we were unable to determine whether such utilization had any impact on subsequent offending or health behaviors.

Policy makers and academic researchers should establish some consensus on what the impact of correctional re-entry programs should be in terms of effects and the duration of such effects. We can then begin to move toward developing quality evaluations of the impacts of evidence-based criminogenic risk assessments, re-entry programs, community services, and communities on the behavior of CJ-involved individuals living in the community. Without such yardsticks against which to measure results, we will continue to lament the rates of recidivism and service follow-through, even though they may be relatively acceptable.

Acknowledgements
The author would like to thank James Keller, JD (Central Florida Progress), Chianta Lindsey, MD, Ms Cindi Burke-Liburd, Mr Bakari Burns (Orange Blossom Family Health Center), Max Wilson, PhD, Earl Hunt (Florida Department of Health), Daniel Bowman (UCF) and the MISTERS staff and participants for their contributions to this study. The results and recommendations contained in this study are those of the authors and do not represent the position of the Florida Department of Health. The author declares no conflicts of interest associated with this work.

Funding

This work was funded by the Florida Department of Health Bureau of HIV/AIDS [grant number 07-009].

References

Akers, T. A., Potter, R. H., & Hill, C. V. (2013). *Epidemiological criminology: A public health approach to crime and violence.* San Francisco, CA: Jossey-Bass.

Andrews, D. A., & Bonta, J. (2010). *The psychology of criminal conduct.* New Providence, NJ: Anderson/Lexis-Nexis.

Anno, B. J. (2001). *Correctional health care: Guidelines for the management of an adequate delivery system.* Washington, DC: US Department of Justice, National Institute of Corrections.

Baillargeon, J., Giordano, T. P., Rich, J. D., Wu, Z. H., Wells, K., Pollock, B. H., & Paar, D. P. (2009). Accessing antiretroviral therapy following release from prison. *JAMA: The Journal of the American Medical Association, 301*, 848–857.

Bayer, R., & Dupuis, L. (1995). Tuberculosis, public health, and civil liberties. *Annual Review of Public Health, 16*, 307–326.

Birgden, A. (2004). Therapeutic jurisprudence and responsivity: Finding the will and the way in offender rehabilitation. *Psychology, Crime & Law, 10*, 283–295.

Blomberg, T. G. (1995). Beyond metaphors: Penal reform as net-widening. In T. G. Blomberg & S. Cohen (Eds.), *Punishment and social control. Essays in honor of Sheldon L. Messinger* (pp. 45–61). New York, NY: Aldine de Gruyter.

Chen, N. E., Meyer, J. P., Avery, A. K., Draine, J., Flanigan, T. P., Lincoln, T., … Altice, F. L. (2011). Adherence to HIV treatment and care among previously homeless jail detainees. *AIDS and Behavior, 17*, 2654–2666. doi:10.1007/s10461-011-0080-2

Cohen, T. H., & Reaves, B. (2007). *Pretrial release of felony defendants in state courts.* Washington, DC: United States Department of Justice, Bureau of Justice Statistics. Retrieved from http://www.ojp.usdoj.gov/bjs/pub/pdf/prfdsc.pdf

Donovan, J. E., & Jessor, R. (1985). Structure of problem behavior in adolescence and young adulthood. *Journal of Consulting and Clinical Psychology, 53*, 890–904.

Frazier, C. E., Richards, P., & Potter, R. H. (1983). Juvenile diversion and net widening: Toward a clarification of assessment strategies. *Human Organization, 42*, 115–122.

Gulliford, M., Figueroa-Munoz, J., Morgan, M., Hughes, D., Gibson, B., Beech, R., & Hudson, M. (2002). What does' access to health care'mean? *Journal of Health Services Research & Policy, 7*, 186–188.

Jessor, R., & Jessor, S. L. (1977). *Problem behavior and psychosocial development: A longitudinal study of youth.* New York, NY: Academic Press.

Lattimore, P. K., & Visher, C. A. (2009). *The multi-site evaluation of SVORI: Summary and synthesis.* Washington, DC: Urban Institute.

Lowenkamp, C. T., & Latessa, E. J. (2005). Increasing the effectiveness of correctional programming through the risk principle: Identifying offenders for residential placement[*]. *Criminology & Public Policy, 4*, 263–290. doi:10.1111/j.1745-9133.2005.00021.x

MacGowan, R., Margolis, A., Richardson-Moore, A., Wang, T., Lalota, M., French, P. T., … Mckeever, J. (2009). Voluntary rapid human immunodeficiency virus (HIV) testing in jails. *Sexually Transmitted Diseases, 36*, S9–S13.

Maruschak, L. M. (2006). *Medical problems of jail inmates.* Washington, DC: Office of Justice Programs.

Maruschak, L. M. (2008). *Medical problems of prisoners.* Washington, DC: Office of Justice Programs.

Potter, R. H., & Rosky, J. W. (2012). The iron fist in the latex glove: The intersection of public health and criminal justice. *American Journal of Criminal Justice, 38*, 276–288.

Reznick, O. G., McCartney, K., Gregorich, S. E., Zack, B., & Feaster, D. J. (2013). An ecosystem-based intervention to reduce HIV transmission risk and increase medication adherence among inmates being released to the community. *Journal of Correctional Health Care, 19*, 178–193. doi:10.1177/1078345813486442

Simpson, D. D., & Knight, K. (2007). Offender needs and functioning assessments from a national cooperative research program. *Criminal Justice and Behavior, 34*, 1105–1112.

Springer, S. A., Pesanti, E., Hodges, J., Macura, T., Doros, G., & Altice, F. L. (2004). Effectiveness of antiretroviral therapy among HIV-infected prisoners: Reincarceration and the lack of sustained benefit after release to the community. *Clinical Infectious Diseases, 38*, 1754–1760.

Stephenson, B. L., Wohl, D. A., Golin, C. E., Tien, H.-C., Stewart, P., & Kaplan, A. H. (2005). Effect of release from prison and re-incarceration on the viral loads of HIV-infected individuals. *Public Health Reports, 120*, 84–88.

Steurer, S. J., Smith, L. G., & Tracy, A. (2001). *Three state recidivism study.* Lanham, MD: Correctional Education Association.

Ward, T., Day, A., Howells, K., & Birgden, A. (2004). The multifactor offender readiness model. *Aggression and Violent Behavior, 9*, 645–673.

Wexler, H. K., & Fletcher, B. W. (2007). National criminal justice drug abuse treatment studies (CJ-DATS) overview. *The Prison Journal, 87*, 9–24.

Wohl, D. A., Scheyett, A., Golin, C. E., White, B., Matuszewski, J., Bowling, M., … Duffin, A. (2011). Intensive case management before and after prison release is no more effective than comprehensive pre-release discharge planning in linking HIV-infected prisoners to care: A randomized trial. *AIDS and Behavior, 15*, 356–364.

Influences on substance use cessation during pregnancy: an exploratory study of women on probation and parole

Rebecca J. Stone and Merry Morash

School of Criminal Justice, Michigan State University, 655 Auditorium Rd, Rm. 560 Baker Hall, East Lansing, MI 48824, USA

Research suggests that a lack of family support, low self-efficacy, mental illness, and life stressors increase the likelihood of women using illicit substances during their pregnancies. These risk factors often characterize the lives of women on probation and parole. The current study uses data from a larger study of women on supervision to explore the risk and protective factors of substance use during pregnancy. Results highlight the importance of self-efficacy, mental health treatment, and family support; and suggest avenues for intervention to improve maternal and infant health outcomes.

The last several decades saw a substantial increase in women under community supervision – a more substantial increase than that for men (Glaze & Bonczar, 2009; Glaze & Parks, 2012). In 2010, there were 712,084 women on probation and 103,374 on parole (Glaze & Parks, 2012). While these numbers have decreased slightly since 2009, women now constitute a greater proportion of the population than in previous decades (Maruschak & Parks, 2012).

The increasing proportion of women under community supervision has serious implications for public health. Between 60 and 80% of incarcerated women are mothers, with approximately 70% of incarcerated women having minor children (Pollock, 2002). These figures are likely to be similar for the population of women on probation and parole, suggesting that many women in this population are of childbearing age. Substance-involved women make up an estimated two-thirds of women offenders (Langan & Pelissier, 2001; Peters, Strozier, Murrin, & Kearns, 1997). Taken together, these characteristics suggest that women on probation and parole may be at increased risk of maternal substance abuse and fetal substance exposure. Though substance use during pregnancy is a phenomenon occurring at every socio-economic level, women who are socially and economically marginalized are more likely to lack the resources necessary to seek treatment and take beneficial health actions to protect themselves and their children. Women on probation and parole are likely to be socially and economically marginalized due to limited employment opportunities, exclusion from welfare benefits and other social services, and restricted access to financial aid for higher education (Allard, 2002; Iguchi, Bell, Ramchand, & Fain, 2005).

Substance use during pregnancy presents a significant risk for both mother and child. The abuse of illicit substances during pregnancy has been linked to poor infant health outcomes. Recent studies conclude that illicit drug use during pregnancy is associated with premature birth, miscarriage, low birth weight, and a variety of behavioral and cognitive problems (Bandstra, Morrow, Mansoor, & Accornero, 2010; Sowell et al., 2010; Velez, Jansson, Schroeder, & Williams, 2009). Pregnant women who use illicit drugs also tend to use alcohol and tobacco, which carry their own risks, and may experience other pregnancy risks, such as poor nutrition, an irregular sleep schedule, or sexually transmitted infection (Sowell et al., 2010). Fearful of being caught, women using substances during pregnancy may engage in risky health behavior to avoid detection. In their qualitative study of women using heroin and stimulants, Murphy and Rosenbaum (1999) found that several women chose to avoid doctors' offices and health clinics. Some women in their study planned unattended births outside of the hospital to avoid drug tests and subsequent involvement with child protection services and the criminal justice system.

It appears that the population of women on probation and parole is at high risk for substance use during pregnancy and the consequential health risks. However, there is a gap in the literature in regard to maternal substance use in the correctional population. Much of the research on substance use and pregnancy occurs in a clinical setting and does not mention the supervision status of women in the sample. To address this gap in the literature, we turned to research on drug use and cessation during pregnancy in other populations to better understand general patterns of drug use during pregnancy and the associated risk and protective factors. In doing so, we set the stage for a unique study of the issue of substance use cessation among pregnant women on probation and parole.

We first examined national statistics on trends in substance use during pregnancy to understand the magnitude of this phenomenon. According to the 2011 *National Survey on Drug Use and Health*, 5% of pregnant women aged 15–44 are current illicit drug users. This rate is higher but not significantly different from the 2008–2009 rate of 4.5%. The rate of current illicit drug use is highest for pregnant women aged 15–17 (20.9%), compared to pregnant women aged 18–25 (8.2%) and 26–44 (2.2%). The overall rate of illicit drug use among pregnant women (5%) is lower than the rate among women who are not pregnant (10.8%), suggesting that many women desist from drug use during their pregnancies (Substance Abuse and Mental Health Services Administration, 2012).

The literature on non-offender populations suggests several risk and protective factors for illicit drug use during pregnancy. Some studies have shown that women with higher levels of educational attainment are less likely to use illicit substances during pregnancy (Abma & Mott, 1991). Ebrahim and Gfroerer (2003) found that drug use during pregnancy was highest among women with less than high school education. Though race is often assumed to be an important predictor of substance use during pregnancy, Chasnoff, Landress, and Barrett (1990) found that rates of positive drug screens for pregnant women were similar for white women (15.4% positive) and black women (14.1%), though black women were reported to health authorities for substance use during pregnancy at a rate approximately 10 times higher than white women.

Just a few studies focus on social and psychological factors that are related to substance use during pregnancy. Mental health issues like stress and depression may lead to some women's continued substance use during pregnancy (Harrison & Sidebottom, 2008; Ockene et al., 2002). Harrison and Sidebottom (2008) also found that lack of transportation predicted drug use continuation throughout pregnancy, though the authors acknowledged that lack of transportation may be a proxy for extreme poverty or social isolation. Women's self-concept as adequate providers for their children has been linked to the cessation of substance use during pregnancy (Massey et al., 2012), though self-concept is likely influenced by other factors mentioned above, such as depression and social isolation.

By identifying predictors of substance use desistance for pregnant women on probation and parole, the present article suggests points of intervention to assist a high-risk group of women in having positive pregnancy outcomes. This approach to developing interventions to reduce barriers to stopping drug use during pregnancy stands in contrast to a trend to criminalize women for using drugs or alcohol during pregnancy (Paltrow, Cohen, & Carey, 2000). Prior research suggests that the criminalization approach can be criticized as unfounded, unjust, and as producing the unintended negative effect of dissuading women from obtaining prenatal care (Lester, Andreozzi, & Appiah, 2004; Poland, Dombrowski, Ager, & Sokol, 1993). In contrast, the present study suggests interventions that have promise for assisting women in the offender population to desist from using substances that may cause fetal harm.

Relevant theoretical constructs

The research described in this article offers a unique contribution by adopting a public health approach to the issue of substance use in pregnancy in a community supervision population. The benefit of the public health approach is that it frames issues as problems to be understood and changed, rather than accepted as inevitable (Mercy, Rosenberg, Powell, Broome, & Roper, 1993). The public health approach emphasizes prevention, evidence-based interventions, and the integration of interdisciplinary efforts by researchers, practitioners, and communities. For the purposes of the present inquiry, we turn to known correlates of substance use cessation to examine their impact on cessation during pregnancy. Public health literature is replete with evidence of the importance of self-efficacy, mental health, and family support to an individual's substance use cessation.

Self-efficacy

Self-efficacy (Bandura, 1977), an individual's perception of his or her capability of performing a particular behavior, is a known predictor of the initiation and maintenance of desistance from substance abuse (Burling, Reilly, Moltzen, & Ziff, 1989; DiClemente et al., 2001; Grella, Hser, Joshi, & Douglas Anglin, 1999; Kadden & Litt, 2011). Self-efficacy has been found to predict coping behavior, level of performance, and perseverance in the face of adversity (Bandura & Locke, 2003). With regard to substance use and addiction, Bandura (1986) notes that people with high self-efficacy are more likely to exert the effort and mobilize the resources needed to resist drinking or drug use and to regard slips or relapses as temporary setbacks rather than unrecoverable failures. Studies have linked self-efficacy to substance use and to treatment outcomes. McKay et al. (2004) examined self-efficacy in a population of patients following residential or outpatient treatment and found that self-efficacy levels were strongly associated with the amount of subsequent substance use and with participation in continuing care. Similarly, Stephens, Wertz, and Roffman (1995) found that self-efficacy predicted post-treatment abstinence and the frequency of subsequent marijuana use. Among patients in residential treatment, higher levels of self-efficacy at treatment discharge are a strong predictor of one-year abstinence. Self-efficacy can also protect against relapse in patients with both substance use and psychiatric disorders (Ramo, Anderson, Tate, & Brown, 2005).

Not all studies provide clear evidence that self-efficacy predicts future abstinence. Dolan, Martin, and Rohsenow (2008) concluded that the effect of self-efficacy may be short-term only, as their study found that higher self-efficacy predicted less drug use three months post-treatment but not after six months. Self-efficacy may be a stronger predictor of desistance from alcohol use than desistance from drug use (Walton, Blow, Bingham, & Chermack, 2003). Furthermore, studies of dual-diagnosis patients (those who have both substance use and mental health disorders) have produced mixed results in regard to self-efficacy and desistance from substance use (Tate et al., 2008; Warren, Stein, & Grella, 2007).

Women on probation and parole are often economically disadvantaged (Morash, 2010) and socially isolated (Rosenbaum, 1989). They are often involved with abusive intimate partners and have histories of family violence and abuse (Batchelor, 2005; Rosenbaum, 1989; Ryder, 2003). Bandura (1977) recognized that psychological processes impact efficacy expectations and that past successes, vicarious experiences, and support and persuasion from others can increase an individual's self-efficacy. This proposition has many implications for women on probation or parole who are trying to desist from substance use during a pregnancy, as these women may have few past successes from which to draw confidence and may lack support from others to spur them into positive behavioral change. Emotional arousal can also impact self-efficacy, and Bandura (1977, p. 198) recognized that 'individuals are more likely to expect success when they are not beset by aversive arousal than if they are tense and viscerally agitated'. Considering the stressful lives of many women on probation and parole (Holtfreter & Morash, 2003; Morash, 2010; Salisbury & Van Voorhis, 2009), it is likely that they are often in states of emotional arousal that undermine positive effects of self-efficacy.

Family support

Family support tends to play a central role in the lives of individuals under supervision of the criminal justice system. Former prisoners may live with family members upon release (Visher, 2007) and rely on family members for material and emotional support (Braman, 2004). Nelson, Deess, and Allen (1999) found that former prisoners consistently cited family support as being an important factor in post-release integration. Bahr, Harris, Fisher, and Harker Armstrong (2010) found that while most participants in their study cited family support as an important resource, unsuccessful parolees reported more conflict with their families than successful parolees. Conflict with family members can lead to stress and frustration, which in turn lead to relapses in substance abuse as a means of coping with negative emotions (Phillips & Lindsay, 2009). One recent study found that higher levels of family conflict coincide with increased odds of drug use after release from prison (Mowen & Visher, 2013). These findings suggest that family support may also play a role in supervised pregnant women's desistance from substance use: women with supportive relationships with their families may face fewer barriers to desistance. We have included a measure of family support in the present inquiry to determine if women with greater family support are more likely than others to desist from substance use during their pregnancies.

Mental health

A study of released prisoners returning to their community found that 34.9% of female study participants self-reported having been diagnosed with a mental health condition (Mallik-Kane & Visher, 2008). Two to three months post-release, 45% of women reported having been diagnosed with a mental health condition. Among those with mental health conditions, 7 of 10 had comorbid substance abuse problems. Data from the National Epidemiologic Survey on Alcohol and Related Conditions suggest that, in the general population, 20% of those suffering from substance use disorders also have one or more mood disorders, and 18% have an anxiety disorder (Grant et al., 2004). Data from the same survey reveal that, among those with drug use disorders, the rates of primary or independent diagnoses of personality, mood, and anxiety disorders are 44, 28, and 24%, respectively (Stinson et al., 2005). In treatment populations, mental health conditions are frequently associated with relapse following drug treatment (Brown, O'Grady, Battjes, & Farrell, 2004; Compton, Cottler, Jacobs, Ben-Abdallah, & Spitznagel, 2003; Norman, Tate, Anderson, & Brown, 2007; Shanahan et al., 2005) and poor program adherence (Hien, Nunes, Levin, & Fraser, 2000). Together, studies of mental health suggest that rates of mental health conditions are likely to be high in populations on probation and parole, and that mental health conditions may interfere with successful cessation of use during pregnancy.

Research purpose

The research reported in this article is unique in that it takes a public health perspective to exploring and making recommendations for encouraging cessation from substance use during pregnancy among women on probation and parole. Specifically, the literature suggests that higher self-efficacy and good relationships with parents influence women to desist from drug use during pregnancy. Mental health problems and severe substance abuse issues appear to promote continued use. This exploratory study identifies which of these factors are non-spurious predictors of cessation for a subgroup of women who are pregnant and who are on probation or parole.

Methodology

Sample and study design

With a secondary analysis of existing data, we consider a subsample of women from a larger study of women on probation and parole. For the larger study, initial interviews were conducted between 1997 and 1999, and follow-up interviews took place approximately 12 months after the initial interview. Data were collected after the beginning of the influx of women into correctional settings, and descriptions of women in the justice system at the time the data were collected and in recent years suggest that female offenders have not changed substantially since the study period (Greenfeld & Snell, 1999; Holtfreter & Morash, 2003; Sarteschi & Vaughn, 2010; Van Voorhis, Salisbury, Wright, & Bauman, 2008).

The original study was designed to compare the experiences of women under traditional types of community supervision with those of women who received supervision geared to addressing gender-related needs. To provide diversity in sample location, data were collected from two counties in a northwestern state and two counties in a midwestern state. During the study period, research staff attempted to sample all women with at least one felony conviction at the start of parole or probation supervision in the four counties. From 1997 to 1999, research staff met with community corrections supervisors to review lists of eligible women beginning probation or parole. Unless the women immediately transferred or could not be contacted for an initial meeting, interviewers met privately with them and invited them to be in the study, after which (if they agreed) the consent process was carried out. A total of 595 women were identified, and 404 (67.9%) took part in an initial interview. Differences between women who did and did not complete the first interview were small; economic offenders without any drug involvement tended not to begin the study, and women with a juvenile record more often took part. Reasons for not completing the first interview included the project staff's inability to make an initial contact, transfer of women out of the county, and refusals. The subsample of women who did participate in the research included 51 women with a recent history of substance use and who were pregnant in the year prior to beginning probation or parole supervision (39 or 76.5%) or during the one-year period of data collection (12 or 23.5%).

Variables

The dependent variable is continuation of drug use during pregnancy, and the two independent variables of interest are self-efficacy and social support. Consistent with the literature reviewed above, other predictors of cessation include mental health and education. Two control variables that might account for outcomes are the seriousness of drug use and the type of probation or parole supervision the women received (i.e. traditional or gender responsive).

Establishing pregnancy and drug use

At the first interview, participants were asked whether they were pregnant at any time in the last year, and in subsequent interviews 6 and 12 months after the first one, this question was repeated for the period since the previous interview. Women responding affirmatively were asked, 'Did you use methadone or any illegal drugs during your pregnancy?' and 'Were you using methadone or any illegal drugs when your baby was born?' In order to determine whether women were on methadone treatment or had used illegal drugs, we used qualitative data from interviews with each woman and case notes from her probation or parole officer. These sources contained information regarding which particular drugs the woman used, the results of urine tests, and information about women's life circumstances around the time of pregnancy. These reports were detailed and provided written information on supervising officers' contact with each woman and her counselors, treatment professionals, and social service providers. The qualitative and quantitative data-sets were compared, and cases with missing or inconsistent information on drug use and pregnancy were dropped to select the subsample of 51 women, 24 who had used illegal drugs during their pregnancies and 27 who had not.

Self-efficacy

The interview schedule contained items from Heppner and Petersen's (1982; Heppner, 1988) Problem Solving Inventory (PSI). In this context, the term 'problem solving' refers to the 'self-directed cognitive-behavioral process by which an individual, couple or group attempts to identify or discover effective solutions for specific problems encountered in everyday living' (D'Zurilla, Nezu, & Maydeu-Olivares, 2004, p. 12). Problem-solving ability is a multidimensional construct consisting of two general components: (1) problem orientation and (2) problem-solving skills (PSS) (D'Zurilla & Goldfried, 1971; D'Zurilla & Nezu, 1982, 1990). Problem orientation is 'a metacognitive process involving the operation of a set of relatively stable cognitive-emotional schemes that reflect a person's general beliefs, appraisals, and feelings about ... his or her own problem-solving ability' (D'Zurilla et al., 2004). This definition is very similar to Bandura's (1995, p. 2) definition of self-efficacy as 'the belief in one's capabilities to organize and execute the courses of action required to manage prospective situations.' The PSI is a 35-item, six-point Likert-style self-report scale designed to measure an individual's perception of his or her problem-solving behavior and attitudes (Heppner & Petersen, 1982). Though Heppner and Petersen's (1982) instrument was derived from the theory of social problem-solving developed by D'Zurilla and Goldfried (1971), it was found to measure constructs not associated with any one theory of social problem-solving.

To remedy this, Maydeu-Olivares and D'Zurilla (1997) conducted a content analysis of the PSI and concluded that two meaningful theoretical constructs can be extracted from the original PSI, (1) problem-solving self-efficacy (PSSE) (i.e. the belief that one is capable of solving problems effectively) and (2) PSS. By selecting the items from the original PSI that most closely approximated these two constructs, Maydeu-Olivares and D'Zurilla (1997) constructed a seven-item PSSE scale and a nine-item PSS scale. For the present analysis, the PSSE scale was used as a measure of self-efficacy, as it most closely resembles the concept as defined by Bandura (1977, 1995). Examples of these items, used in conjunction with a Likert rating scale, are: 'When my first try to solve a problem fails, I feel I can't handle the situation' (reverse coded) and 'Given enough time and effort, I believe I can solve most problems that I have.' Following Maydeu-Olivares and D'Zurilla (1997) recommendation, we recoded the appropriate PSI items so that higher scores indicate high confidence in problem-solving efficacy. The resultant seven-item scale served as our measure of self-efficacy (Cronbach's $\alpha = .80$).

Family support

Responses to the following question were used to indicate parental support in the present analysis: 'Do you have a poor relationship with your parents?' Women answered either yes or no. This was the best available indicator of family support.

Mental illness

Mental health is measured by a five-item scale (Cronbach's $\alpha = .75$). The items used to construct this scale are 'Have you ever been evaluated by a psychologist/psychiatrist?' 'Have you ever been an in-patient in a mental health hospital or program?' 'Are you currently under the care of a psychologist/psychiatrist?' 'Prior to this program, have you ever been prescribed drugs for treating a mental health issue?' and 'Have you ever attempted suicide?' Affirmative answers were coded 1 and the items were summed to produce the scale. Scores ranged from 0 to 5 with a mean of 1.53 (SD = 1.47).

Substance abuse

The severity of each respondent's substance use was determined by a seven-item scale (Cronbach's $\alpha = .84$). This scale consists of the items 'Have drugs ever been a problem?', 'Has alcohol ever been a problem?', 'Did you ever break the law while under the influence of drugs or alcohol?', 'Did drugs or alcohol ever cause any marital of family problems?', 'Have you ever had problems in school or at work because of drugs or alcohol?', 'Have you ever suffered from loss of control because of drug or alcohol use?', and 'Have you ever suffered from loss of control from drug or alcohol use such as drinking or taking drugs until unconsciousness (black outs) or sneaking drinks or drugs?' Possible responses were yes and no, and the sum was viewed as a count of indicators, with more indicators reflecting greater severity. Total scores ranged from 0 to 7, with a mean of 3.76 (SD = 2.39).

Education

The education measure consists of five categories for the highest level of education completed by the participant: sixth through ninth grade, 10th or 11th grade, completion of high school or a GED program, technical school or some college, and a four-year undergraduate degree or more. Education was used rather than income to indicate socio-economic status because education is more resistant to change. Specifically, a woman who was highly educated before spending time in prison may be released on parole and struggle to find work, resulting in a low income, but her educational attainment will not change.

Supervision style

Type of programming is not a central focus of the present research. However, the original study was designed to compare women receiving gender responsive and traditional types of probation and parole supervision. For women who were pregnant during the one-year study, programming could influence whether they desisted from substance use during pregnancy. Indeed, for the full sample interviewed for the original study, women with gender responsive supervision reported statistically significantly higher levels of a supervising officer or treatment professional checking to see if they had needs related to pregnancy, substance use, mental health, domestic violence, or general health. They also reported statistically significantly higher levels of referrals or direct help for substance use, mental health, and domestic violence. Of the 51 women considered in the present analysis, more (24 or 66.7% vs. 17 or 33.3%) were in the gender responsive than traditional types of probation and parole. Since type of programming may affect desistance from drug use for the women who were pregnant during the year of supervision, the type of supervision (gender responsive or traditional) was included as a control variable in multivariate analyses to predict whether pregnant women continued to use drugs or did not.

Missing data

Very little data were missing for the variables of interest. Two women were missing some responses for the self-efficacy scale and another two women were missing responses to questions used to compute the mental health scale. One woman was missing a response used for the substance abuse scale, and another was missing the measure of family support. For all other variables, no data were missing. Because the missing data appeared to be missing at random, values were imputed with LISREL software's multiple imputation procedure, which predicted the missing value from other variables considered in the analysis as well as correlated variables not included in analysis (age and a score reflecting level of risk).

Analysis

Bivariate analysis was used to compare women who did and did not desist from drug use on the several quantitative measures of independent variables and the control variable. Logistic regression was then used to determine which relationships remained significant while controlling for other variables, and to determine which independent variables were the strongest predictors. The size of the odds ratio is not sufficient for determining which of the significant variables is the strongest predictor of substance use during pregnancy. To allow for a comparison of the strength of different predictors in the model, the regression coefficients were standardized. Partially standardized logit coefficients were calculated using the formula:

$$\beta_j^* = \frac{\beta_j \sigma_j}{\sigma_d}, j = 1, \ldots, k,$$

where β_j^* is the standardized coefficient, σ_j is the standard deviation of x_j, and σ_d is the standard deviation of the disturbance term ε in the latent model for the continuous variable (Allison, 1999; DeMaris, 2004). Because ε has a standard logistic distribution, its standard deviation is $\frac{\pi}{\sqrt{3}} = 1.8138$.

Results

Description of the sample and bivariate comparison

Of the 51 women in the subsample, 24 continued their drug use while pregnant and 27 did not. Their average age was 26.4 years, and there was no significant difference in age between the groups (for those who desisted, $x = 26.4$, SD $= 6.0$; for those who continued, $x = 26.4$, SD $= 5.3$; $t = -.006$, df $= 49$, $p = .995$). The subsample consisted of women who identified as white/Caucasian (35, 68.6%), black/African-American (10, 19.6%), Native American or Indian (4, 7.8%), and other or multiple races (2, 3.9%). The desisters and non-desisters did not differ significantly in racial composition ($\chi^2 = 4.15$, df $= 3$, $p = .245$). For education, 41.2% (21) of women in the sample had graduated from high school or earned a

GED and 37.3% (19) had less education. The remaining 21.6% (11) had attended a technical school or completed some college courses. There was no significant difference between the two groups in the level of education achieved ($\chi^2 = .45$, df $= 3$, $p = .930$).

Bivariate analysis

Bivariate analysis was conducted to determine the relationship of each independent variable to women's continuation or desistence from substance use during pregnancy. Both self-efficacy and mental health were found to be significantly associated with substance use during pregnancy in the expected directions. The group of women who desisted from substance abuse had a higher mean score on the PSSE scales and a lower mean score on the mental health scale. The other variables of interest were not significant at this level of analysis (Table 1).

Multivariate analysis

Collinearity diagnostics were examined for the current analyses. Correlations, variance inflation factors, tolerance, and condition index values were all at acceptable levels, indicating that multicollinearity is not a problem.

The regression model results show that the level of education, the severity of the substance abuse problem and the program style of the probation or parole office (gender-responsive or traditional) are not significant predictors of women's continuation of drug use during pregnancy. The severity of mental health issues and the presence of a good relationship with her parents approach significance but do not break the .05 threshold. Holding all else constant, the only significant predictor is scores on the PSSE scale ($p = .04$), indicating that women with higher self-efficacy scores are significantly less likely than women with lower scores to continue their drug use throughout their pregnancies. The measures of mental health and family support approach significance but do not break the .05 threshold. These results, though they do not achieve significance, are in the expected directions. If this same analysis were to be conducted on a larger sample, it is possible that the mental health and family support measures would be significant in the model. Women who

Table 1. Bivariate analysis to compare persisters and desisters.

Independent variable	Means and standard deviations		t	p
	Desisters ($n = 27$)	Persisters ($n = 24$)		
PSSE	35.74 (3.79)	31.25 (7.37)	2.69	.01
Mental health	.70 (1.14)	1.92 (1.56)	−3.20	.00
Severity of substance abuse	3.18 (2.72)	4.42 (1.79)	−1.93	.06
Family support*	.78 (.42)	.52 (.51)	1.91	.06
Type of supervision*	.67 (.48)	.67 (.48)	.00	1.00
Education**			.45	.93
Grades 6–9	3 (11.1%)	2 (8.3%)		
Grade 10 or 11	8 (29.6%)	6 (25.0%)		
Grade 12 or GED	10 (37.0%)	11 (45.8%)		
Technical school/some college	6 (52.9%)	5 (20.8%)		

*$0 = $ no, $1 = $ yes. **χ^2.

have better relationships with their parents are less likely to continue using drugs throughout their pregnancies. Women with higher scores on the mental health scale (indicating poorer mental health) are more likely to continue their drug use throughout their pregnancies. Had the mental health scale achieved significance, the partially standardized coefficient indicates that it would be the strongest predictor of drug use during pregnancy. As it stands, only the measure of PSSE achieved significance in this model (Table 2).

Discussion

The purpose of this research was to increase understanding of desistance from drug use during pregnancy in a sample of women on probation and parole. The analysis revealed that high self-efficacy was a significant predictor of desistance. This relationship was significant even when controlling for other known correlates of drug use persistence in pregnancy, including mental health problems and family support.

Although the data available for analysis allowed us to take a first step in exploring substance use cessation during pregnancy for a correctional population, the nature of the data resulted in limitations. First, the sample size is small. Substance use during pregnancy is a very sensitive topic and not easy to study without deliberately targeting this hidden population. Of the more than 400 women in the original sample, only 51 had been pregnant in the past year *and* had valid information indicating substance involvement. Only 24 could be identified as having persisted with their drug use during their pregnancies. There were likely other women in the larger sample who had used substances during a pregnancy at some point in their lives, but as this topic was not the focus of the original study, this information was not captured. Second, the questions only detect whether illegal substances were used at *any* time during the pregnancy and do not detect behavioral changes *during* the pregnancy. Finally, the study design precludes determination of how each woman's self-efficacy is impacted by her changing life circumstances or by any

Table 2.   Results of logistic regression analysis.

	B	S.E.	p^{*}	Exp. (B)	Partially standardized coefficients
Constant	3.99	3.14	.203	54.35	–
PSSE	−.15	.07	.036	.86	−.07
Mental health	.54	.28	.054	1.72	.52
Family support	−1.67	.86	.051	.19	−.17
Gender-responsive supervision	.39	.79	.621	1.49	.32
Education	.11	.39	.782	1.12	.07
Severity of substance abuse	.21	.18	.266	1.23	.14
N	51				
Cox and Snell R^2	.35				
−2 Log likelihood	47.71				
Model χ^2	21.29				
	($p = .002$)				

*Values rounded to the third decimal place to demonstrate that though the values for mental health and family support round to .05, they do not break the .05 threshold.

treatment programs she may be attending. We statistically controlled for the type of supervision women received, but this is likely insufficient to fully control for the influence of external stressors, different treatment programs, and individual probation and parole officers' interactions with women on their caseloads.

Although caution is required in drawing firm conclusions, the study results suggest that interventions to increase women's self-efficacy may decrease the likelihood of maternal substance use and fetal drug exposure. Relevant to the design of interventions, some studies have identified specific activities that promote changes in self-efficacy. Active participation in goal-setting (Lozano & Stephens, 2010), skills-building activities (Ilgen, McKellar, & Moos, 2007), and coping skills training (Roffman & Stephens, 2005) have all been found to increase self-efficacy and lead to avoidance and resistance to drug use. Skills training exercises include homework practice exercises tailored to individuals' high-risk situations (Annis, Schober, & Kelly, 1996). The homework assignments should, as suggested by Bandura (1986), be challenging, require a moderate degree of effort, require little external aid, and be relevant to the problem situations the individual frequently encounters. The assignments should function by increasing the perception of personal control in problem situations, and success in the assignments should reflect on the individual's improved performance. Past success and performance accomplishments are a principle source of efficacy beliefs (Bandura, 1986), suggesting that small achievements in homework assignments may provide valuable support to individuals when they are faced with real problem situations.

Despite the promise of interventions to increase self-efficacy, it is important to recognize that more research is needed on such interventions. A review of the literature on self-efficacy in the substance abuse field found that few substance abuse treatments were specifically designed to increase self-efficacy (Kadden & Litt, 2011). Instead, self-efficacy has typically been examined as an afterthought in treatment outcome studies. For example, one review found that 7 of 10 studies measuring self-efficacy pre- and post-intervention reported positive effects on self-efficacy, but the interventions varied so broadly that it was not possible to identify the best programs for enhancing self-efficacy (Hyde, Hankins, Deale, & Marteau, 2008).

Further research is also needed to demonstrate the interconnections of self-efficacy with mental health and family support. Though mental health and family support did not break the threshold of significance in the present analysis, these variables may still be important predictors of successful drug use desistance during pregnancy. The design of the current study (i.e. the lack of longitudinal data and the relatively small sample size) does not allow for an examination of the relationship between self-efficacy, family support and mental health, though many other studies suggest that these three are closely related. Minimizing depressive symptoms has been found to increase self-efficacy (Dolan et al., 2008; McKellar, Ilgen, Moos, & Moos, 2008). Poor relationships with family members may also contribute to both poor mental health and low self-efficacy. It is possible that a woman's family might disapprove of her drug use and distance themselves from her, leading to a breakdown in their relationship and ability to provide encouragement and support for her desistance from drugs. It is also possible that that a woman's relationship with her family was already poor prior to her pregnancy or the onset of her drug use, and that this poor relationship played some role in influencing her path towards her eventual probation or parole supervision. Bandura (1994) recognizes that early self-efficacy experiences are centered in the family, and that parents who are responsive to their infants and encourage exploratory play and the healthy development of language skills can instill greater self-efficacy in their children. Women whose families of origin are characterized as disruptive, disorganized, and violent are unlikely to have had these early life experiences to promote their self-efficacy. In this case, young women may rely on peers for the development of their self-knowledge, but negative peer relationships can stunt the growth of self-efficacy. These negative relationships may cause women to withdraw from social interaction and experience a lowered sense of self-worth, decreasing their likelihood of believing they can overcome life obstacles. This isolation may lead to depression, anxiety, or other mental health issues. Future qualitative research as well as quantitative, longitudinal research with an adequately sized sample would be useful for establishing the potentially complex ways that self-efficacy, family support, mental health, and other factors are related to substance use desistance during pregnancy.

Based on the present study as well as the existing literature, it appears that the most successful treatment approach would meet women's needs for social support and mental health treatment while increasing their self-efficacy. Wraparound-style treatment programs that include methods to increase self-efficacy may be effective. Wraparound models can be more effective than traditional approaches because they address the multiple needs of women on probation and parole in a coordinated and comprehensive manner. They facilitate women's access to multiple services within their communities, for example by providing medical services, social support services (e.g. housing or employment assistance), HIV/AIDS testing, mental health counseling and treatment, transportation services, child care, and other types of help (Greenfield et al., 2007; Reed & Leavitt, 2000). The wraparound approach, which the National Institute of Drug Abuse (2012) recommends for substance abuse treatment, allows for women's needs to be met in a coordinated way rather than in a piecemeal fashion that leaves women constantly struggling (Covington & Bloom, 2003).

Treatment approaches such as those discussed so far stand in stark contrast to the criminal justice approach, which emphasizes detection and punishment of drug-using pregnant women. Pointing to an unintended consequence of the criminal justice approach, in their review of the literature, Banwell and Bammer (2006) describe the construction of a deviant risk group that stigmatizes mothers seeking treatment for substance use. They argue that the construction of the risk category of substance-using women pits the health and welfare of young children against the behaviors (and failures) of their mothers, who are considered only to the extent that they transmit harms to their children (2006, p. 505). Substance-using mothers and pregnant women are considered part of a higher risk category than other women and may be placed under heightened surveillance by health and welfare professionals, increasing the likelihood that they will suffer consequences ranging from subtle discrimination to child removal and arrest (Boyd, 1999; Murphy & Rosenbaum, 1999; Paltrow, 1999). Fear of these consequences represents a significant barrier to care for mothers and pregnant women, with many mothers reporting that they delayed or avoided prenatal care altogether out of fear of punishment (Murphy & Rosenbaum, 1999; Poland et al., 1993; Roberts & Nuru-Jeter, 2010; Roberts & Pies, 2010). This result has unwanted consequences, since substance-using women who *do* receive prenatal care experience more positive birth outcomes and have greater opportunities for other health promoting interventions than women who do not receive care (Berenson, Wilkinson, & Lopez, 1996; El-Mohandes et al., 2003; Green, Silverman, Suffet, Taleporos, & Turkel, 1979; MacGregor, Keith, Bachicha, & Chasnoff, 1989; Racine, Joyce, & Anderson, 1993; Richardson, Hamel, Goldschmidt, & Day, 1999).

The arguments in favor of punitive policies suggest that if women are sufficiently afraid of punishment, they will find a way to change. In contrast, Bandura (1990, p. 11) espouses a 'shift in emphasis from trying to scare people into healthy behavior to empowering them with the tools for exercising personal control over their health habits.' A public health approach rather than criminal justice apprehension thus seems justified.

There is a great need for further research on substance use and pregnancy for correctional populations. Qualitative studies are needed to illuminate the context of the findings presented here. For example, more detailed description of the family relationships classed as 'good' and 'bad' may provide more clues for possibly interventions or treatments to promote maternal and infant health. Similarly, more focused inquiry into the relationship of self-efficacy to substance use during pregnancy may reveal some treatment options that are more promising than others or describe connections between self-efficacy, substance use, mental health, and family relations. More specific questions about the timing of substance use and pregnancy, the types of substances used, and the inclusion of measures of alcohol and tobacco use are also important for future research and theory development. The present study should be considered as a starting point on the path to a better understanding of prenatal substance use among women on probation and parole.

References

Abma, J. C., & Mott, F. L. (1991). Substance use and prenatal care during pregnancy among young women. *Family Planning Perspectives, 23*, 117–128.

Allard, P. (2002). *Life sentences: Denying welfare benefits to women convicted of drug offenses.* Washington, DC: The Sentencing Project.

Allison, P. (1999). *Logistic regression using SAS: Theory and application.* Cary, NC: SAS Institute.

Annis, H. M., Schober, R., & Kelly, E. (1996). Matching addiction outpatient counseling to client readiness for change: The role of structured relapse prevention counseling. *Experimental and Clinical Psychopharmacology, 4*, 37–45.

Bahr, S. J., Harris, L., Fisher, J. K., & Harker Armstrong, A. (2010). Successful reentry: What differentiates successful and unsuccessful parolees? *International Journal of Offender Therapy and Comparative Criminology, 54*, 667–692.

Bandstra, E. S., Morrow, C. E., Mansoor, E., & Accornero, V. H. (2010). Prenatal drug exposure: Infant and toddler outcomes. *Journal of Addictive Diseases, 29*, 245–258.

Bandura, A. (1977). Self-efficacy: Toward a unifying theory of behavioral change. *Psychological Review, 84*, 191–215.

Bandura, A. (1986). *Social foundations of thought and action: A social cognitive theory.* Englewood Cliffs, NJ: Prentice-Hall.

Bandura, A. (1990). Perceived self-efficacy in the exercise of control over AIDS infection. *Evaluation and Program Planning, 13*, 9–17.

Bandura, A. (1994). Self-efficacy. In V. S. Ramachaudran (Ed.), *Encyclopedia of human behavior* (pp. 71–81). New York, NY: Academic Press.

Bandura, A. (1995). *Self-efficacy in changing societies.* Cambridge: Cambridge University Press.

Bandura, A., & Locke, E. A. (2003). Negative self-efficacy and goal effects revisited. *Journal of Applied Psychology, 88*, 87–99.

Banwell, C., & Bammer, G. (2006). Maternal habits: Narratives of mothering, social position and drug use. *International Journal of Drug Policy, 17*, 504–513.

Batchelor, S. (2005). 'Prove me the bam!': Victimization and agency in the lives of young women who commit violent offenses. *The Journal of Community and Criminal Justice, 52*, 358–375.

Berenson, A. B., Wilkinson, G. S., & Lopez, L. A. (1996). Effects of prenatal care on neonates born to drug-using women. *Substance Use and Misuse, 31*, 1063–1076.

Boyd, S. C. (1999). *Mothers and illicit drugs: Transcending the myths.* Toronto: University of Toronto Press.

Braman, D. (2004). *Doing time on the outside: Incarceration and family life in urban America.* Ann Arbor: University of Michigan Press.

Brown, B. S., O'Grady, K., Battjes, R. J., & Farrell, E. V. (2004). Factors associated with treatment outcomes in an aftercare population. *American Journal on Addictions, 13*, 447–460.

Burling, T. A., Reilly, P. M., Moltzen, J. O., & Ziff, D. C. (1989). Self-efficacy and relapse among inpatient drug and alcohol abusers: A predictor of outcome. *Journal of Studies on Alcohol, 50*, 354–360.

Chasnoff, I. J., Landress, H. J., & Barrett, M. E. (1990). The prevalence of illicit-drug or alcohol use during pregnancy and discrepancies in mandatory reporting in Pinellas County, Florida. *New England Journal of Medicine, 322*, 1202–1206.

Compton, W. M., Cottler, L. B., Jacobs, J. L., Ben-Abdallah, A., & Spitznagel, E. L. (2003). The role of psychiatric disorders in predicting drug dependence treatment outcomes. *American Journal of Psychiatry, 160*, 890–895.

Covington, S., & Bloom, B. (2003). Gendered justice: Women in the criminal justice system. In B. Bloom (Ed.), *Gendered justice: Addressing female offenders.* Durham, NC: Carolina Academic Press.

DeMaris, A. (2004). *Regression with social data: Modeling continuous and limited response variables.* Hoboken, NJ: John Wiley & Sons.

DiClemente, C. C., Carbonari, J. P., Daniels, J. W., Donovan, D. M., Bellino, L. E., & Neavins, T. M. (2001). *Project MATCH hypotheses: Results and causal chain analyses* (pp. 239–257). NIH Publication No. 01-4238. Bethesda, MD: National Institute on Alcohol Abuse and Alcoholism.

Dolan, S. L., Martin, R. A., & Rohsenow, D. J. (2008). Self-efficacy for cocaine abstinence: Pretreatment correlates and relationship to outcomes. *Addictive Behaviors, 33*, 675–688.

D'Zurilla, T., & Nezu, A. (1982). Social problem solving in adults. In P. C. Kendall (Ed.), *Advances in cognitive–behavioral research and therapy* (pp. 201–274). New York, NY: Academic Press.

D'Zurilla, T., Nezu, A., & Maydeu-Olivares, A. (2004). Social problem solving: Theory and assessment. In E. C. Chang, T. D'Zurilla, & L. Sanna (Eds.), *Social problem solving: Theory, research, and training* (pp. 11–27). Washington, DC: American Psychological Association.

D'Zurilla, T. J., & Goldfried, M. R. (1971). Problem solving and behavior modification. *Journal of Abnormal Psychology, 78,* 107–126.

D'Zurilla, T. J., & Nezu, A. M. (1990). Development and preliminary evaluation of the social problem-solving inventory. *Psychological Assessment, 2,* 156–163.

Ebrahim, S. H., & Gfroerer, J. (2003). Pregnancy-related substance use in the United States during 1996–1998. *Obstetrics and Gynecology, 101,* 374–379.

El-Mohandes, A., Herman, A. A., Nabil El-Khorazaty, M., Katta, P. S., White, D., & Grylack, L. (2003). Prenatal care reduces the impact of illicit drug use on perinatal outcomes. *Journal of Perinatology, 23,* 354–360.

Glaze, L. E., & Bonczar, T. P. (2009). *Probation and parole in the United States, 2008.* Washington, DC: Bureau of Justice Statistics.

Glaze, L. E., & Parks, E. (2012). *Correctional populations in the United States, 2011.* Washington, DC: Bureau of Justice Statistics.

Grant, B. F., Stinson, F. S., Dawson, D. A., Chou, S. P., Dufour, M. C., Compton, W., … Kaplan, K. (2004). Prevalence and co-occurrence of substance use disorders and independent mood and anxiety disorders. *Archives of General Psychiatry, 61,* 807–816.

Green, M., Silverman, I., Suffet, F., Taleporos, E., & Turkel, W. V. (1979). Outcomes of pregnancy for addicts receiving comprehensive care. *The American Journal of Drug and Alcohol Abuse, 6,* 413–429.

Greenfield, S. F., Brooks, A. J., Gordon, S. M., Green, C. A., Kropp, F., McHugh, R. K., … Miele, G. M. (2007). Substance abuse treatment entry, retention, and outcome in women: A review of the literature. *Drug and Alcohol Dependence, 86*(1), 1–21.

Greenfeld, L., & Snell, T. (1999). *Women offenders (No. NCJ 175688).* Washington, DC: Bureau of Justice Statistics, US Department of Justice.

Grella, C. E., Hser, Y. I., Joshi, V., & Douglas Anglin, M. (1999). Patient histories, retention, and outcome models for younger and older adults in DATOS. *Drug and Alcohol Dependence, 57,* 151–166.

Harrison, P. A., & Sidebottom, A. C. (2008). Alcohol and drug use before and during pregnancy: An examination of use patterns and predictors of cessation. *Maternal and Child Health Journal, 13,* 386–394.

Heppner, P. (1988). *The Problem Solving Inventory.* Palo Alto, CA: Consulting Psychologist Press.

Heppner, P., & Petersen, C. H. (1982). The development and implications of a personal problem-solving inventory. *Journal of Counseling Psychology, 29,* 166–175.

Hien, D. A., Nunes, E., Levin, F. R., & Fraser, D. (2000). Posttraumatic stress disorder and short-term outcome in early methadone treatment. *Journal of Substance Abuse Treatment, 19,* 31–37.

Holtfreter, K., & Morash, M. (2003). The needs of women offenders. *Women and Criminal Justice, 14,* 137–160.

Hyde, J., Hankins, M., Deale, A., & Marteau, T. M. (2008). Interventions to increase self-efficacy in the context of addiction behaviours: A systematic literature review. *Journal of Health Psychology, 13,* 607–623.

Iguchi, M., Bell, J., Ramchand, R., & Fain, T. (2005). How criminal system racial disparities may translate into health disparities. *Journal of Health Care for the Poor and Underserved, 16,* 48–56.

Ilgen, M., McKellar, J., & Moos, R. (2007). Personal and treatment-related predictors of abstinence self-efficacy. *Journal of Studies on Alcohol and Drugs, 68,* 126–132.

Kadden, R. M., & Litt, M. D. (2011). The role of self-efficacy in the treatment of substance use disorders. *Addictive Behaviors, 36,* 1120–1126.

Langan, N., & Pelissier, B. (2001). Gender differences among prisoners in drug treatment. *Journal of Substance Abuse, 13,* 291–301.

Lester, B. M., Andreozzi, L., & Appiah, L. (2004). Substance use during pregnancy: Time for policy to catch up with research. *Harm Reduction Journal, 1,* 1–44.

Lozano, B. E., & Stephens, R. S. (2010). Comparison of participatively set and assigned goals in the reduction of alcohol use. *Psychology of Addictive Behaviors, 24,* 581–591.

MacGregor, S. N., Keith, L. G., Bachicha, J. A., & Chasnoff, I. J. (1989). Cocaine abuse during pregnancy: Correlation between prenatal care and perinatal outcome. *Obstetrics and Gynecology, 74,* 882–885.

Mallik-Kane, K., & Visher, C. (2008). *Health and prisoner reentry: How physical, mental, and substance abuse conditions shape the process of reintegration.* Washington, DC: Urban Institute.

Maruschak, L. M., & Parks, E. (2012). *Probation and parole in the United States, 2011.* Washington, DC: Bureau of Justice Statistics.

Massey, S. H., Neiderhiser, J. M., Shaw, D. S., Leve, L. D., Ganiban, J. M., & Reiss, D. (2012). Maternal self concept as a provider and cessation of substance use during pregnancy. *Addictive Behaviors, 37,* 956–961.

Maydeu-Olivares, A., & D'Zurilla, T. (1997). The factor structure of the Problem Solving Inventory. *European Journal of Psychological Assessment, 13,* 206–215.

McKay, J. R., Foltz, C., Leahy, P., Stephens, R., Orwin, R. G., & Crowley, E. M. (2004). Step down continuing care in the treatment of substance abuse: Correlates of participation and outcome effects. *Evaluation and Program Planning, 27,* 321–331.

McKellar, J., Ilgen, M., Moos, B. S., & Moos, R. (2008). Predictors of changes in alcohol-related self-efficacy over 16 years. *Journal of Substance Abuse Treatment, 35,* 148–155.

Mercy, J. A., Rosenberg, M. L., Powell, K. E., Broome, C. V., & Roper, W. L. (1993). Public health policy for preventing violence. *Health Affairs, 12,* 7–29.

Morash, M. (2010). *Women on probation and parole: A feminist critique of community programs and services.* Boston, MA: Northeastern University Press.

Mowen, T. J., & Visher, C. A. (2013). Drug use and crime after incarceration: The role of family support and family conflict. *Justice Quarterly,* 1–23. Published online February 27.

Murphy, S., & Rosenbaum, M. (1999). *Pregnant women on drugs.* New Brunswick, NJ: Rutgers University Press.

National Institute on Drug Abuse. (2012). *Principles of drug abuse treatment for criminal justice populations: A research-based guide* (pp. 1–36). No. 11-5316. Rockville, MD: National Institutes of Health.

Nelson, M., Deess, P., & Allen, C. (1999). *The first month out: Post-incarceration experiences in New York City.* New York, NY: The Vera Institute.

Norman, S. B., Tate, S. R., Anderson, K. G., & Brown, S. A. (2007). Do trauma history and PTSD symptoms influence addiction relapse context? *Drug and Alcohol Dependence, 90,* 89–96.

Ockene, J., Ma, Y., Zapka, J., Pbert, L., Valentine Goins, K., & Stoddard, A. (2002). Spontaneous cessation of smoking and alcohol use among low-income pregnant women. *American Journal of Preventive Medicine, 23,* 150–159.

Paltrow, L. M. (1999). Pregnant drug users, fetal persons, and the threat to Roe V. Wade. *Albany Law Review, 62,* 999–1055.

Paltrow, L. M., Cohen, D. S., & Carey, C. A. (2000). *Year 2000 overview: Governmental responses to pregnant women who use alcohol or other drugs.* Women's Law Project and the National Advocates for Pregnant Women. Retrieved from http://www.csdp.org/news/news/gov_response_review.pdf

Peters, R. H., Strozier, A. L., Murrin, M. R., & Kearns, W. D. (1997). Treatment of substance-abusing jail inmates. Examination of gender differences. *Journal of Substance Abuse Treatment, 14,* 339–349.

Phillips, L. A., & Lindsay, M. (2009). Prison to society: A mixed methods analysis of coping with reentry. *International Journal of Offender Therapy and Comparative Criminology, 55,* 136–154.

Poland, M. L., Dombrowski, M. P., Ager, J. W., & Sokol, R. J. (1993). Punishing pregnant drug users: Enhancing the flight from care. *Drug and Alcohol Dependence, 31,* 199–203.

Pollock, J. M. (2002). *Women, crime, and prison.* Belmont, CA: Wadsworth.

Racine, A., Joyce, T., & Anderson, R. (1993). The association between prenatal care and birth weight among women exposed to cocaine in New York City. *JAMA: The Journal of the American Medical Association, 270,* 1581–1586.

Ramo, D. E., Anderson, K. G., Tate, S. R., & Brown, S. A. (2005). Characteristics of relapse to substance use in comorbid adolescents. *Addictive Behaviors, 30,* 1811–1823.

Reed, B., & Leavitt, M. (2000). Modified wraparound and women offenders in community corrections: Strategies, opportunities and tensions. In M. McMahon (Ed.), *Assessment to assistance: Programs for women in community corrections* (pp. 1–106). Lanham, MD: American Correctional Association.

Richardson, G. A., Hamel, S. C., Goldschmidt, L., & Day, N. L. (1999). Growth of infants prenatally exposed to cocaine/crack: Comparison of a prenatal care and a no prenatal care sample. *Pediatrics, 104,* e18.

Roberts, S. C. M., & Nuru-Jeter, A. (2010). Women's perspectives on screening for alcohol and drug use in prenatal care. *Women's Health Issues, 20,* 193–200.

Roberts, S. C. M., & Pies, C. (2010). Complex calculations: How drug use during pregnancy becomes a barrier to prenatal care. *Maternal and Child Health Journal, 15,* 333–341.

Roffman, R. A., & Stephens, R. S. (2005). Relapse prevention for cannabis abuse and dependence. In G. A. Marlatt & D. M. Donovan (Eds.), *Relapse prevention: Maintenance strategies in the treatment of addictive behaviors* (pp. 179–207). New York, NY: Guilford Press.

Rosenbaum, J. (1989). Family dysfunction and female delinquency. *Crime and Delinquency, 35,* 31–44.

Ryder, J. (2003). *Antecedents of violent behavior* (Unpublished doctoral dissertation). City University of New York, New York.

Salisbury, E. J., & Van Voorhis, P. (2009). Gendered pathways: A quantitative investigation of women probationers' paths to incarceration. *Criminal Justice and Behavior, 36,* 541–566.

Sarteschi, C. M., & Vaughn, M. G. (2010). Double jeopardy: A review of women offenders' mental health and substance abuse characteristics. *Victims and Offenders, 5,* 161–182.

Shanahan, C. W., Lincoln, A., Horton, N. J., Saitz, R., Winter, M., & Samet, J. H. (2005). Relationship of depressive symptoms and mental health functioning to repeat detoxification. *Journal of Substance Abuse Treatment, 29,* 117–123.

Sowell, E. R., Leow, A. D., Bookheimer, S. Y., Smith, L. M., O'Connor, M. J., Kan, E., … Thompson, P. M. (2010). Differentiating prenatal exposure to methamphetamine and alcohol versus alcohol and not methamphetamine using tensor-based brain morphometry and discriminant analysis. *Journal of Neuroscience, 30,* 3876–3885.

Stephens, R. S., Wertz, J. S., & Roffman, R. A. (1995). Self-efficacy and marijuana cessation: A construct validity analysis. *Journal of Consulting and Clinical Psychology, 63,* 1022–1031.

Stinson, F. S., Grant, B. F., Dawson, D. A., Ruan, W. J., Huang, B., & Saha, T. (2005). Comorbidity between DSM-IV alcohol and specific drug use disorders in the United States: Results from the National Epidemiologic Survey on Alcohol and Related Conditions. *Drug and Alcohol Dependence, 80,* 105–116.

Substance Abuse and Mental Health Services Administration. (2012). *Results from the 2011 National Survey on Drug Use and Health: Summary of national findings* (No. NSDUH Series H-44, HHS Publication No. (SMA) 12-4713). Rockville, MD: Author.

Tate, S. R., Wu, J., McQuaid, J. R., Cummins, K., Shriver, C., Krenek, M., & Brown, S. A. (2008). Comorbidity of substance dependence and depression: Role of life stress and self-efficacy in sustaining abstinence. *Psychology of Addictive Behaviors, 22,* 47–57.

Van Voorhis, P., Salisbury, E., Wright, E. J., & Bauman, A. (2008). *Achieving accurate pictures of risk and identifying gender responsive needs: Two new assessments for women offenders.* Washington, DC: US Department of Justice, National Institute of Corrections.

Velez, M. L., Jansson, L. M., Schroeder, J., & Williams, E. (2009). Prenatal methadone exposure and neonatal neurobehavioral functioning. *Pediatric Research, 66,* 704–709.

Visher, C. (2007). Returning home: Emerging findings and policy lessons about prisoner reentry. *Federal Sentencing Reporter, 20,* 93–102.

Walton, M. A., Blow, F. C., Bingham, C. R., & Chermack, S. T. (2003). Individual and social/environmental predictors of alcohol and drug use 2 years following substance abuse treatment. *Addictive Behaviors, 28,* 627–642.

Warren, J. I., Stein, J. A., & Grella, C. E. (2007). Role of social support and self-efficacy in treatment outcomes among clients with co-occurring disorders. *Drug and Alcohol Dependence, 89,* 267–274.

Moving prison health promotion along: towards an integrative framework for action to develop health promotion and tackle the social determinants of health

James Woodall[a], Nick de Viggiani[b], Rachael Dixey[a] and Jane South[a]

[a]School of Health and Wellbeing, Leeds Metropolitan University, G08 Queen Square House, Leeds LS2 8AF, UK; [b]Faculty of Health and Life Sciences, Department of Health and Applied Social Sciences, University of the West of England, Bristol BS16 1DD, UK

The majority of prisoners are drawn from deprived circumstances with a range of health and social needs. The current focus within 'prison health' does not, and cannot, given its predominant medical model, adequately address the current health and well-being needs of offenders. Adopting a social model of health is more likely to address the wide range of health issues faced by offenders and thus lead to better rehabilitation outcomes. At the same time, broader action at governmental level is required to address the social determinants of health (poverty, unemployment and educational attainment) that marginalise populations and increase the likelihood of criminal activities. Within prison, there is more that can be done to promote prisoners' health if a move away from a solely curative, medical model is facilitated, towards a preventive perspective designed to promote positive health. Here, we use the Ottawa Charter for health promotion to frame public health and health promotion within prisons and to set out a challenging agenda that would make health a priority for everyone, not just 'health' staff, within the prison setting. A series of outcomes under each of the five action areas of the Charter offers a plan of action, showing how each can improve health. We also go further than the Ottawa Charter, to comment on how the values of emancipatory health promotion need to permeate prison health discourse, along with the concept of salutogenesis.

Context

There is now a wealth of evidence that demonstrates that people in prison face a disproportionate burden of health and social inequality. Many diseases, illnesses and long-term conditions are over-represented in prison populations and disadvantaged social circumstances are commonplace for most of those imprisoned. For these reasons, some have argued that public health and health promotion in the prison population is as much, if not more, significant than efforts in the 'free' community (Ross, 2013); yet, the concept and practice of public health and health promotion in prison is both contested and underdeveloped with significant variation in its application in prison systems globally. This paper outlines what the authors regard as 'prison health' and what the determinants of prison health are. Our argument is that a social model of health in prison has not been taken far enough, and that and an appreciation of the wider social determinants of health has not been fully addressed in terms of policy responses.

Our view stands in stark contrast to the 'bounded' medical model which usually prevails in prison health systems, and that regards health as being an absence of disease. The paper explores whether our understanding of a social model of prison health can lead to a workable framework to develop policy and practice for public health and health promotion in prison. Moreover, we suggest how this framework may be measured and what may constitute successful outcomes. We do not claim to provide startlingly new contributions, but we do wish to move the health promoting prison agenda along by reigniting debate. Thus, we also discuss how the determinants of health agenda can be developed into one concerned with the *social determination* of health – that is health being determined by 'the people'. Prisons do not enable prisoners to take control of the factors governing their health, and where health promotion has been developed, it tends to be within a medical model of health promotion, focussing on individual lifestyle 'choices'. Examples are where education about alcohol or drugs is provided, without full understanding of the social context or of enabling offenders to develop skills in avoiding substance misuse on the outside or inside. Further, given the reoffending rates, prisons are not rehabilitative institutions and the criminal justice system as it operates appears unable to tackle the social conditions that lead to initial offending or reoffending.

The contribution of the World Health Organisation

It is important to discuss the contribution to date made to public health and health promotion in prison by the World Health Organisation (WHO), as their strategic oversight has been a salient factor in ensuring that prison health is on the public health agenda of various nations (Gatherer, Moller, & Hayton, 2005). We offer this as a brief overview to those who may not be aware of efforts in this area to date.

The work developed by WHO Europe has been particularly prominent (Moller, Gatherer, & Dara, 2009; Møller, Stöver, Jürgens, Gatherer, & Nikogosian, 2007) and is seen as a model to enable global expansion. The American Public Health Association's human rights committee, for example, is working to bring the lessons learned from successful European prison health initiatives to the Americas (Anonymous, 2008). Designated work in other WHO regions is less apparent and tends to 'lag' behind policy developments in Europe. This is not to say that public health and health promotion work is not present in these regions, rather it is not coordinated as clearly under the WHO banner. Current guidance from the WHO suggests that the health promoting prison is underpinned by four key pillars and grounded in a 'settings approach' – the premise of which is that investments in health are made in social institutions whose primary remit is not health (Dooris, 2007). These four key pillars acknowledge that prisons should be: safe, secure, reforming and health promoting; and grounded in the concept of decency and respect for human rights (Hayton, 2007).

Equivalence is a further principle that informs public health efforts in prison. The principle of 'equivalence' is based on the view that individuals detained in prison must have the benefit of care equivalent to that provided to the general public (Niveau, 2007). Critics have argued, however, that an equivalent health service in prison is an 'insufficient public health response' (Lines, 2006, p. 276) given the extent of health and social inequalities.

The WHO has been active in publishing key documents and statements to shape global public health efforts in prison, including: 'Mental Health Promotion in Prisons' (WHO, 1998), 'HIV in Prisons' (WHO, 2001a), 'Prisons, Drugs and Society' (WHO, 2001b), 'Promoting the Health of Young People in Custody' (WHO, 2003) and a practical guide to the essentials in prison health (WHO, 2007). In 2005, Gatherer et al. (2005) appraised the progress made by the WHO in prisons and concluded that despite considerable achievements, formidable barriers remained including overcrowding and unhygienic facilities, rising prison populations, inherent traditions, political perspectives and the reluctance of staff to evolve their ways of working and resource restrictions. Indeed, whilst the concept of a health promoting prison seems laudable, prisons are not primarily geared to improving health (Smith, 2000). In short, Awofeso (2010) lists the issues as:

(1) The concentration of unhealthy individuals;
(2) The amplification of unhealthy behaviours;
(3) The deterioration of existing health conditions;
(4) The dissemination of infectious diseases and
(5) Post-release morbidity and mortality, resulting from health conditions developed or exacerbated during incarceration.

We would add that loss of freedom in itself is inherently pathogenic and whilst prisons have a duty of care to prisoners they also must place to the fore concerns with public safety and thus with prison security.

What is prison health?

While recognising that prisoners are not a homogenous group, epidemiological assessment of the population shows undeniable health need, with research evidence consistently demonstrating that the prevalence of ill health is higher than reported in the wider community (Senior & Shaw, 2007). Mental health problems (Fazel & Danesh, 2002; WHO, 2008), long-standing physical disorders (Plugge, Douglas, & Fitzpatrick, 2006; Stewart, 2008) and drug and alcohol issues (Social Exclusion Unit, 2002; The Centre for Social Justice, 2009; Woodall, 2012) are commonplace. In addition to health problems, multifaceted social issues face the prison population which in turn impact on health (Rutherford & Duggan, 2009; Stewart, 2008). Jacobs back in 1977 observed how the prison population was influenced by social trends and processes beyond the prison wall (Jacobs, 1977). Indeed, many of those entering the criminal justice system have experienced a lifetime of social exclusion, including poor educational backgrounds, low incomes, meagre employment opportunities, lack of engagement with normal societal structures, low self-esteem and impermanence in terms of accommodation (including bouts of homelessness) and relationships with family members (Department of Health, 2009; Levy, 2005; Prison Reform Trust, 2009; Senior & Shaw, 2007; Social Exclusion Unit, 2002).

Developing clear strategies to address the health and social issues reported in the prison population relies on how health is defined. The concept of 'prison health' has, in the main, been clearly aligned to a biomedical perspective

(Sim, 1990). Morris and Morris (1963, p. 193), in their study of Pentonville prison, encapsulated the predominant discourse which surrounded prison health:

> For the prison, health is essentially a negative concept; if men are not ill, de facto they are healthy. While most modern thinking in the field of social medicine has attempted to go further than this, for the prison medical staff it is not an unreasonable operational definition.

In the American correctional system, the concept of health had been underpinned in a similar way. When the Medical Centre for Federal Prisoners in Springfield was opened in 1933, it was 'dedicated solely' to caring for the diseased and the 'broken bodies and minds of offenders' (Bosworth, 2002, p. 79). Through this lens, health is conceptualised in a reductionist, rather than holistic, way and viewed in terms of pathology, disease, diagnosis and treatment (Warwick-Booth, Cross, & Lowcock, 2012). This has notable implications, as health is defined by its absence of disease and not the attainment of positive health and well-being. More-over, the medical model of health tends to focus on physical dimensions of health (such as physical fitness and functionality) rather than mental (such as having a sense of purpose and meaning) and social dimensions of health (such as feeling connected to the community).

Anno's (2004) comparative article reviewing US prison health services in the 1970s to the present argues that while much has been done to improve health systems in prison the focus remains on addressing acute physical and mental medical need, rather than addressing other dimensions of prisoners' health and well-being. Moreover, an international systematic review (which included studies from Australasia, Europe, US and Africa) conducted by Herbert, Plugge, Foster, and Doll (2012) concluded that prison health services fail to fully exploit public health and 'upstream' health promotion work. This has been echoed in England and Wales where critical reviews of prison health services described a reactive and inefficient service, underpinned by a medical model that was largely blind to the social determinants of health and thus failed to exploit public health opportunities (HMIP, 1996).

There have been clear efforts in recent times to detach prison health services from the biomedical perspective (Department of Health, 2002; HM Prison Service, 2003) with US commentators like Winterbauer and Diduk (2013) arguing that public health efforts in prison have now evolved from simply disease-based models. Baybutt, Hayton, and Dooris (2010) have optimistically argued that the medical model of health provision has been reformed; however, the discourse surrounding health in prison keeps its heavy, unbalanced focus on disease control, eradication, screening and testing. In contrast, the social model sees ill-health as caused by social conditions and thus the solution lies in tackling those underlying social causes of poor health, including low levels of literacy, poor interpersonal skills, lack of employability skills, social exclusion and so on. This recognition of social factors remains side-lined in policy and practice discourse.

Previous research has raised questions about the definitions of health currently deployed in the prison environment and how 'normative' health need, i.e. that defined by expert/professional opinion, has governed much prison health policy and planning (Smith, 2002). Arguably, the social model of health encompasses 'lay' perspectives about health, taking into account subjective experience and understandings. Indeed, Robertson (2006) suggests that lay perceptions have been influential in supporting a cultural shift away from a biomedical perspective towards a more holistic and integrated understanding of health and well-being. Whilst research on prisoners' lay health views is scanty, it does demonstrate that factors such as access to the outdoors and social relationships, especially contact with family members, were intimately intertwined with prisoners' ideas around being healthy (Woodall, 2010b). Bosworth, Campbell, Demby, Ferranti, and Santos (2005) have noted that it can be difficult, without serving a sentence, to know what prison life is like; yet, this understanding is vital if we are to address 'health' in a meaningful way. The extent that this broader understanding of 'health' and well-being can be incorporated into prison health strategy is debatable given the current concern overwhelmingly remaining with disease prevention and management rather than with an acknowledgement of the broader social determinants of health and of lay perspectives on what constitutes health.

The determinants of prisoner health

Public health and health promotion interventions within prison settings have been consistently criticised because they frequently focus on the symptoms of the problem rather than tackling the root causes of poor health, such as the social determinants of health (Caraher et al., 2002). Marquart, Merianos, Hebert, and Carroll's (1997) conceptual framework for prison public health was a starting-point that usefully demonstrated the interaction of prisoners' pre-prison health conditions, the impact on health caused by admission to prison and the impact during imprisonment. More recently, and drawing on a similar school of thought, de Viggiani (2006) has argued that both deprivation and importation factors are significant health determinants within prison. This framework delineates those factors caused by imprisonment that contribute to ill health (deprivation) and those which are a result of circumstances pre-dating a custodial sentence (importation). Smith (2000) suggests that health problems experienced by prisoners are entrenched in their wider environment and their experience of inequality, poverty and disadvantage. She notes that public health attempts in prison contribute towards dealing with behaviour change, but it is only when the collective factors that produce ill-health (outside prison) are tackled, will there be any real health improvement. This is reiterated by Caraher et al. (2002) who suggest that there is a need for health promotion in prison, but also for wider public policy which addresses the broader determinants of health and illness.

The imported nature of individuals' pre-existing health issues to the prison setting was inferred by Goffman (1968, p. 12) who suggested that inmates come into the institution with a 'presenting culture' derived from their 'home world'. In other words, an individual imports life experiences into the prison which may influence their health. As an example, 32% of the prison population are homeless prior to their incarceration and over two-thirds of prisoners are unemployed prior to imprisonment (Social Exclusion Unit, 2002). Both of these social circumstances are known to impact on physical, mental and social components of health. It can be argued, however, that prison itself is also harmful to health. Regardless of an individual's background prior to incarceration, the prison can inflict ill health onto those who are placed there through the deprivation of liberty. Gresham Sykes (1958) in his classic study of a maximum security prison, suggested that imprisonment itself was painful and that it deprived individuals not only of their physical liberty, but goods and services, heterosexual relationships, autonomy and security.

These deprivations collectively threatened the prisoner's personality and sense of personal worth. As an example, cell confinement has a deleterious effect on health, particularly for those with pre-existing mental health issues (Shalev, 2008). As a further example, overcrowded prison systems have implications for the transmission of communicable disease and for potentially limiting prisoners' access to services and support due to low staff-prisoner ratios. Perhaps more implicit are the influences within prison that are clearly detrimental to all facets of a prisoner's health and well-being. As an example, studies show that many prisoners are motivated to stop smoking, but often increase the number of cigarettes they smoke in prison to cope with the 'suffocating boredom' of prison life (Belcher, Butler, Richmond, Wodak, & Wilhelm, 2006; Lester, Hamilton-Kirkwood, & Jones, 2003; Sim, 2002; Squires & Measor, 2001). The literature also suggests that bullying (Edgar, O'Donnell, & Martin, 2003; Ireland, 2002; Ireland & Ireland, 2000), violence (Edgar et al., 2003; Lahm, 2009; Reyes, 2001), homophobia (Gear, 2007; Hensley, 2000; Newton, 1994) and racism (Bhui, 2009; Spalek, 2002; Spencer, Haslewood-Pocsik, & Smith, 2009) still remains in modern prison systems.

A persuasive argument is for a more integrative conceptual model, whereby a combination of the deprivations of prison life and importation of pre-prison circumstances contribute to prisoner health. However, in their current guise, prison policy remains focussed on individually centred lifestyle interventions or disease prevention activities and there remains an oversimplification of the determinants influencing prisoners' health. As an example, the English and Welsh Prison Services' strategy for promoting health focuses on smoking, healthy eating and nutrition and healthy lifestyle (HM Prison Service, 2003). In terms of addressing health, there is an overemphasis on individual behaviour to the exclusion of broader social and structural processes that are at work both in prison and wider society. Through this lens, poor health rests with the individual, with the prison setting simply functioning as a neutral vehicle offering favourable circumstances to undertake individually focused health activities. We argue that a more radical, upstream and holistic outlook is required and we advocate for a shift away from a purely expedient view which considers the prison as a convenient venue for addressing the health lifestyles of offenders.

The promulgation of health should be integral to the institution's culture and this includes considering architecture, policies, ethos, social structures, prisoner-staff relationships and how these impact on individuals. This suggests that enduring change can only reasonably happen when the emphasis moves away from individual behaviour to changes at social and structural levels (de Viggiani, 2007). Thus, in tandem with the interventions within prison, action needs to be taken to address the deprived and pathogenic environments that the majority of prisoners were brought up in and to which they inevitably return upon release. This will require prisons to work more collaboratively with agencies in the community and while this poses challenges, they are not insurmountable as shown by Lincoln, Miles, and Scheibel's (2007) discussion on collaborations across organisations working within and outside the prison system. Moreover, Visher and Travis (2003) argue that the research and academic community also need to target more efforts to understand how best to manage the prison-community transition that offenders face.

A prison health action and outcomes framework

Our argument is that to address the health and social inequalities faced by the prison population, a broader social model of health and an appreciation of wider determinants is necessary. However, by adopting such a holistic philosophy it 'opens up' a range of possible influences on health and this can be challenging for policy-makers and for practitioners whose aim is that of public health improvement in prison settings. In short, can our understanding of a social model of prison health lead to a workable framework to develop policy and practice for the improved health of prisoners?

For the remainder of the paper, we attempt to offer an overarching prison health action and outcomes framework to guide policy, practice and evaluation. This is particularly useful, given that there are few models which indicate how healthy prison settings can be achieved (Ross, 2013). Our framework is informed by the Ottawa Charter, an influential health promotion strategy document emerging in 1986, which indicated that 'health' is wider than 'healthcare' and that health educa-tion alone cannot bring about improved health (WHO, 1986). The Charter attempts to address both structural forces that influence health (e.g. policy, environment) and also the individual health choices (agency) that people make (Rütten & Gelius, 2011). The Charter provides five principal areas for action: building healthy public policy, creating supportive environments; strengthening community action, develop-ing personal skills, reorientating health services (WHO, 1986). These five areas have continued to provide a useful framework for the delivery of health promotion and public health programmes (Kickbusch, 2003) and authors claim that the Charter has had a *'phenomenal influence'* on the development of health promotion practice over the past two decades (Nutbeam, 2008, p. 436). Despite this endorsement, the explicit application of the Charter to prison settings has been rarely considered (although see Ramaswamy & Freudenberg, 2007; Woodall & South, 2012).

Given the diversity of health issues in the prison setting, we have applied each of the five principal areas for action within the Ottawa Charter. Moreover, we have attempted to capture some of potential outcomes and where possible the links between changes in personal, social and environmental factors, intermediate health outcomes, such as health behaviours, and longer term health and social outcomes (Nutbeam, 1998).

Building healthy public policy

Building healthy public policy can be seen as the chief innovation of the Ottawa Charter moving health promotion firmly away from an individual, lifestyle focus and towards those actions which could impact upon whole populations. No smoking policies, for example, or polices governing minimum nutritional standards for institutional food automatically create potential for healthier outcomes without individuals needing to decide to take healthier actions. Thus, Kemm (2001) argues that healthy public policy is any policy that increases the health and well-being of those individuals that it affects. Policy can occur at an institutional level within an organisation (e.g. prison) or at a macro-level (e.g. national policy).

Certain policy at the institutional (prison) level can be at odds with the goals of healthy public policy. For example, being locked and confined within a prison cell can be detrimental to physical and mental health (Shalev, 2008; Woodall, 2010a). However, a goal should be that institutional policies are considered in relation to the impact on prisoners' health and should be designed to ensure that 'healthy choices are easier choices' (Kickbusch, 1986; Milio, 1986). As an example, condom availability in Australian prisons is not consistent across states, but Butler and colleagues (Butler, Richters, Yap, & Donovan, 2013) reported that condoms were more likely to be used in prisons where policies allowed condoms to be freely available. As the authors noted, this may be hardly surprising; however, it demonstrates that where healthy choices are easy to make, it results in better health choices.

At the macro-level, it is unrealistic to suggest that the prison setting with its limited resources and capacity can address the issue of poor prisoner health in isolation. Certainly prisons have a contribution to make, but they are only one component in a very complex jigsaw. One major way in which the multifaceted health and social issues surrounding offenders' lives will be resolved is when the unequal distribution of power in society is redistributed and wider social inequalities (e.g. poverty, unemployment) are addressed through macro-policy interventions. This has been reiterated by several other scholars, including Link and Phelan who have consistently argued that societal interventions are needed to produce major health benefits for populations (Link & Phelan, 2002; Phelan, Link, & Tehranifar, 2010). Their theory of fundamental causes is particularly apt when considering the health of prison populations. Indeed, St Leger (1997, p. 101) suggests that when adopting a healthy setting (i.e. prison) there is a requirement to always stay with 'the big picture'. If released prisoners, for instance, are to refrain from reengaging with drugs and find secure accommodation and employment then this is ultimately contingent upon effective social policy (Knepper, 2007). Dooris (2007, 2009), therefore, encourages advocates and public health professionals within settings to 'connect upwards' to ensure that broader political, economic and social factors are being addressed through political advocacy:

Connecting upwards: A focus on the importance of settings programmes and initiatives working upwards, using advocacy and mediation to ensure action on the underlying determinants of health that may lie outside of their boundaries or immediate remit. (Dooris, 2007, p. 139)

Outcomes which may demonstrate progress at an institutional level in terms of building healthy public policy may include:

- Prisons operating at their correct occupational levels.
- Appropriate staff-prisoner ratios.
- Prisoners having adequate time out of their cell.
- Meaningful occupation provided in prison that has application to employment post-release.
- All prisoners being allocated a personal officer for pastoral support.
- Prison catering that meets nutritional standards.
- Sufficient contact with family.

At a macro-level, positive outcomes include:

- An increased number of prisoners finding suitable accommodation on release.
- Prisoners gaining employment, education and training opportunities in the community on their release.
- Reduced reoffending.

Creating supportive environments

A focus on creating supportive environments emphasises the importance of 'place' and shows how this is inextricably bound to health. Creating healthier prisons requires establishing prison environments that address the physical and social environments of the setting (Ramaswamy & Freudenberg, 2007) and this includes considering architecture, prison policies, structures, prisoner-staff relationships and how these impact on individuals.

Two short examples show how the prison environment can influence health. First, prison overcrowding has both direct and indirect health outcomes (Ross, 2013). Disease transmission, for example, may be a direct effect but issues such as increased violence and prisoner unrest may also be a secondary adverse health outcome. Second, evidence shows that a prisoner's mental health is often contingent on regular family visits (Woodall, Dixey, Green, & Newell, 2009). However, prison visits have generally declined over the past number of years (Broadhead, 2002; Salmon, 2005) and one explanation for this is that families entering prison can be treated unsympathetically by staff (Broadhead, 2002).

Selected outcomes that demonstrate positive health outcomes through addressing the prison environment include:

- Reduced overcrowding.
- Reduced violence.
- Increased opportunities for meaningful occupation.
- Improved access to prison facilities (e.g. library and gymnasium).
- Preserved or improved family bonds.
- Improved prisoner – prison staff relationships.
- Better access to services.

Strengthening community action

Strengthening community action is defined in the Ottawa Charter as:

> ... effective community action in setting priorities, making decisions, planning strategies and implementing them to achieve better health. At the heart of this process is the empowerment of communities, their ownership and control of their own endeavours and destinies. (WHO, 1986, p. iv)

Whilst empowering prisoners has never been an accepted pursuit in prison systems, even regarded as 'morally questionable and politically dangerous' (The Aldridge Foundation & Johnson, 2008, p. 2), there is a growing recognition that contemporary prisons should be 'supportive and empowering' (de Viggiani, Orme, Powell, & Salmon, 2005, p. 918). One example now commonly seen in prisons in England and Wales is the formation of prison councils to provide prisoners with democratic participation in prison life (Edgar, Jacobson, & Biggar, 2011). These councils allow prison representatives to comment and shape policy and practices in the prison as well as suggesting recommendations for action (Solomon & Edgar, 2004). Moreover, in recent times formal peer interventions have also become an integral feature of prison life and have continued to be driven, in part, by an active citizenship in prisons agenda (Edgar et al., 2011). Evidence from international peer-based schemes show prisoners feeling able to discuss issues and be listened to and leading to improvements in prison culture (South et al., forthcoming), which in turn creates more supportive environments. This harnesses the mutual support often naturally and informally developed between prisoners and further mitigates the development of hostile, bullying cultures which are so detrimental to health and well-being.

There are clear benefits when prisoners are able to participate and articulate their views; most notably, it can improve prisoners' self-esteem, improve the running of institutions and can improve staff – prisoner relationships (Solomon & Edgar, 2004). Despite this, Levenson and Farrant (2002) note that participation is rarely intrinsic to prison cultures. Indeed, where prisoner involvement has emerged it is often sporadic and uneven and not consistent across the prison estate (Solomon, 2004; Solomon & Edgar, 2004).

Selected outcomes that demonstrate strengthened community action in a prison setting may include:

- Prisoners' active involvement in institutional planning and strategy development.
- Reduced demands on prison staff as a result of a cadre of trained prison peer-workers.
- Improved prison ethos and culture leading to increased well-being, reduced stress for both inmates and staff, reduced violence.

Developing personal skills

The acquisition of personal skills is imperative for people to have control over their health, and this applies equally to prisoners. The development of personal skills conceivably constitutes a myriad of possibilities, but centres on the need to provide information and education for health, enhance life skills and influence health beliefs and values (Dixey, Cross, Foster, & Woodall, 2013). Many interventions under the rubric of developing personal skills in prison have adopted a harm-reduction or risk-reduction philosophy using educational approaches. This philosophy aims to prevent or reduce negative health effects associated with certain types of behaviour (WHO, 2005). For example, a harm-reduction programme for women offenders in the US (Lehma, 2001) showed positive results in terms of improvements in knowledge and self-efficacy of participants in relation to the prevention of hepatitis and sexually transmitted infection. However, personal skills may also include providing practical skills training in life and social skills, such as parenting courses, like those described by Jarvis, Graham, Hamilton, and Tyler (2004).

Peer interventions in the prison settings also show promising results in developing prisoners' personal skills, including improvements in prisoners' knowledge of HIV (Bryan, Robbins, Ruiz, & O'Neill, 2006; Collica, 2002; Ross, Harzke, Scott, McCann, & Kelley, 2006; Scott, Harzke, Mizwa, Pugh, & Ross, 2004) and uptake of HIV testing (Zack, Smith, Andrews, & May, 2013), knowledge of sexually transmitted infections (Sifunda et al., 2008), beliefs, intentions and reported increases in condom use (Bryan, et al., 2006; Grinstead, Zack, Faigeles, Grossman, & Blea, 1999; Magura, Kang, & Shapiro, 1994) and increased inclination to practice safer drug using behaviours (Collica, 2002).

Although not exhaustive, outcomes that demonstrate changes to prisoners' personal skills at an individual level include:

- Improved knowledge and awareness.
- Changes in attitudes and beliefs.
- Improved self-efficacy.
- Communication and listening skills.
- Behavioural intentions.
- Reductions in risk behaviour.

System level outcomes may include:

- Reduced transmission rates.
- Greater uptake of services.

Reorienting health services

The final area addressed by the Ottawa Charter is that health care services need to consider their health promotion potential and to embrace preventive approaches as well as the usual curative emphasis. Health services should not merely be seen as the place to go when someone is ill or has a health problem, but rather, as a place where they also go to become more well and to get advice on staying healthy. Freudenberg's (2001) review of the effect of good health promotion practices within US prisons shows that it *can* impact positively on the health of communities, particularly those poorer urban communities from which the majority of prisoners are drawn.

Health services have reoriented to some extent in primary health care on the 'outside' but this shift may not have fully permeated the prison health care service yet. Thus Whitehead (2006, p. 123) suggested that prison nurses, 'must first embrace the radical health promotion reforms that are emerging from the current literature', if they are to keep up with contemporary needs and a newer ethos. Meanwhile, Awofeso (2005) has suggested that prison health care could be made more efficient by focusing on health promotion, including more preventive services and restructuring staffing. Back in 1996, Squires (1996) argued that the problem in the UK was more than simply who commissioned prison health services, and that non-health professional and agencies outside prisons needed to be included in order to change institutional cultures both within health services and the prison.

A further challenge under this area of action is to educate people to use health services appropriately and in a timely fashion. As the majority of prisoners globally are men, and much is known about men's health care-seeking behaviours, (for instance, White and Johnson (2000) explore men's delay in seeking help for chest pain, and Buckley and Ó Tuama (2010) describe Irish men's behaviours as consumers of health care), there is much that could be achieved in terms of health education and patient education for prisoners so that they know how and when to access appropriate health care both inside prison and upon release.

Outcomes that would demonstrate a reorientation of health services would include:

- More emphasis on positive health within prison health care.
- A greater understanding of preventive approaches among health care staff.

- Better understanding of signs and symptoms among prisoners and thus earlier help seeking.
- Development of a socio-ecological model of health promotion as opposed to one focused on individual lifestyle and behaviour change alone.

Moving beyond the Ottawa charter

Whilst the Ottawa charter remains the foundation for health promotion, it is more than 25 years since it was written. Health promoters were heartened by the WHO's Commission on the Social Determinants of Health (Marmot, Friel, Bell, Houweling, & Taylor, 2008) which quite rightly turned a focus on the 'causes of the causes', something that health promotion has long highlighted. It could be argued that the WHO's Commission on the Social Determinants of Health shows some continuity with the biomedical approach to disease and ill-health, showing the continued dominance of the latter in the discourse. Certainly in various national government reports and those from the UN concerning determinants there is a real emphasis on the proximate causes of ill health, those related to individual lifestyles, 'choices' and 'risk factors'. Thus the 'causes of the causes' discourse, resonating with Link and Phelan's theory of fundamental causes, has perhaps become rhetorical rather than being revolutionary.

Emancipatory health promotion has citizenship and personal agency at its heart, enabling individuals and communities to change the material circumstances in which they live, and this relates back to the original and much-quoted definition of health promotion used in the Ottawa Charter. Emancipatory health promotion thus prioritises the *social determination* of health, not simply the *social determinants* of health. However, there seems to be a great disjuncture between the ideas embedded within emancipatory health promotion, with its emphasis on empowerment and people taking control of the factors determining their health, and the reality on the ground facing those experiencing health inequalities, especially those imprisoned. Health inequalities mean that people bear the scars of social conditions in their bodies and minds, as demonstrated by data showing higher rates of a range of disease amongst those from 'lower' social classes. 'Embodiment' is an outward show of power differentials, though those scars are often carried internally, in the form of social alienation, depression, despair, low expectations and criminality. As noted, offenders are drawn disproportionately from more deprived social strata. It would be naive to suggest that prisons can prioritise empowerment of prisoners, as the main purpose of prison is punishment through loss of liberty and to keep the public safe. However, if prisons are to prevent reoffending, and also to address health, there needs to be a push to see how far they can take on more of the key principles of 'emancipatory health promotion'.

However, as Woodall, Dixey, and South (2013, p. 7) say in a paper that explores how key elements of health promotion discourse – choice, control and implicitly, empowerment – are contradictory and puzzling in the context of health promoting prison settings:

> Empowerment is central to becoming the author of one's own life and being able to control the forces that exist in pathogenic and criminogenic environments. The paradox is that prisons are by their nature disempowering yet are tasked with creating more empowered individuals capable of taking control of their lives on release.

In other words, as most prisoners are expected to be released at some point and to not only move away from their previously criminal life but also to take control of the pathogenic circumstances which caused it, they need to be equipped to exercise some agency, control and choice. However, these opportunities to exercise agency and control will be constrained whilst 'inside'. Prisoners' lives have often been systematically regimented and controlled (by the prison regime) that their ability to cope with choices and responsibilities in the community is diminished. How, therefore, can health be socially determined by prisoners and other offenders, given that the *social determination* of health requires citizens to have a voice, power and skills? Can prison settings be 'salutogenic'? This is the real challenge to 'prison health' in the twenty first century.

The concept of salutogenesis has perhaps been more well developed in the Scandinavian countries than elsewhere, and Servan (2012), discussing successful reintegration of women prisoners in Norway, has argued that 'This approach (salutogenesis) provides insights that more traditional studies on recidivism and desistance is not able to give.' Allies in related areas such as design and architecture are also calling to move health improvement further up the prison agenda: 'All new prison design policies should include health impact assessments, and prison design should be modified accordingly' (Awofeso, 2011). The Halden prison in Norway is perhaps the most well-known example of a prison designed to be more humane, with health improvement an explicit goal. There are an increasing number of examples of community-based health promotion initiatives that have been adopted within prison settings. These should be welcomed as they often provide prisoners with the responsibility that underpins meaningful citizenship and successful rehabilitation back into society. Indeed, we can think of people in prison in two discrete ways – as 'citizens in prison' or as prisoners (Svensson, 1996). A contemporary prison system, embracing the values of health promotion, should embrace the former rather than the latter and equip individuals with the necessary skills to reintegrate successfully back into society. Prisoners often wish to take control and make choices which are beneficial for their own health and rehabilitation and yet systemic barriers can inhibit such decisions. Conditions in the prison setting must empower prisoners through offering responsibilities, choice and control over *their* long-term rehabilitation process rather than deskilling and disempowering those who are imprisoned.

Conclusions

Our philosophical stance on 'prison health' is embedded in a social model that moves away from a reductionist, biomedical focus to a viewpoint whereby health is influenced by a range of factors that can be structural and environmental in nature. This position poses challenges to those working in prison health services as it suggests that prisoners' health is influenced by countless factors which lie outside the health workers' control. However, we argue that health is the concern of all those working within the prison, and not only that of the dedicated 'health' staff. Indeed, the essence of a healthy setting is that every aspect of that institution is carefully scrutinised in order to maximise its health potential.

It makes sense to health promoters to use the Ottawa Charter to frame an agenda for improvement in prison health, as the Charter is widely recognised to be as useful and relevant as a basis for public health and health promotion in the twenty-first century as it was when first developed (Nutbeam, 2008; Sparks, 2011). By drawing on the action areas of the Ottawa Charter (WHO, 1986), this paper has outlined a feasible framework to develop policy and practice for the health promoting prison that rests on a social model. The five action areas are overlapping and inter-related and should not be seen as mutually exclusive. The paper attempts to outline what outcomes of success within a social model of prisoner health may constitute, although we acknowledge that these are by no means exhaustive and that guidance has not been offered on how these outcomes may be measured. We also suggest that there are contradictions within emancipatory health promotion especially in relation to offender populations. It is difficult to see how poorer communities can be fully empowered, with power structures subverted, let alone how incarcerated groups could be. Prison health promotion thus needs to be realistic in terms of what it can achieve but what it must do is take into account the socio-economic conditions, the real material situation and the structures of power in which criminogenic behaviour is generated.

Developing prison-based public health and health promotion is not easy and those who are currently working to deliver successful interventions in this setting are doing so within an environment of paradoxical values and philosophies. Approaches to health, particularly health promotion, *have* developed considerably within prisons but there is still a way to go. We hope that the framework presented here offers those working in the field an opportunity to reflect on current practice and to consider prisoners' health in a more holistic sense that recognises that health is more than just the absence of disease.

References

Anno, B. J. (2004). Prison health services: An overview. *Journal of Correctional Health Care, 10*, 287–301.

Anonymous. (2008). Advocates working to improve prison health in the Americas. *The Nation's Health, 38*, 4.

Awofeso, N. (2005). Making prison health care more efficient. *British Medical Journal, 331*, 248–249.

Awofeso, N. (2010). Prisons as social determinants of hepatitis C virus and tuberculosis infections. *Public Health Reports, 125*, 25–33.

Awofeso, N. (2011). Disciplinary architecture: Prison design and prisoners' health. *Hektoen International: A Journal of Medical Humanities, 3*, 1–4.

Baybutt, M., Hayton, P., & Dooris, M. (2010). Prisons in England and Wales: An important public health opportunity? In J. Douglas, S. Earle, S. Handsley, L. Jones, C. Lloyd, & S. Spurr (Eds.), *A reader in promoting public health. Challenge and controversy* (2nd ed., pp. 134–142). Milton Keynes: Open University Press.

Belcher, J. M., Butler, T., Richmond, R. L., Wodak, A. D., & Wilhelm, K. (2006). Smoking and its correlates in an Australian prisoner population. *Drug and Alcohol Review, 25*, 343–348.

Bhui, H. S. (2009). Prisons and race equality. In H. S. Bhui (Ed.), *Race and criminal justice* (pp. 83–101). London: Sage.

Bosworth, M. (2002). *The US federal prison system*. Thousand Oaks, CA: Sage.

Bosworth, M., Campbell, D., Demby, B., Ferranti, S. M., & Santos, M. (2005). Doing prison research: Views from inside. *Qualitative Inquiry, 11*, 249–264.

Broadhead, J. (2002). Visitors welcome – Or are they. *The New Law Journal, 152*, 7014–7015.

Bryan, A., Robbins, R. N., Ruiz, M. S., & O'Neill, D. (2006). Effectiveness of an HIV prevention intervention in prison among African Americans, Hispanics, and Caucasians. *Health Education & Behavior, 33*, 154–177.

Buckley, J., & Ó Tuama, S. (2010). 'I send the wife to the doctor'– Men's behaviour as health consumers. *International Journal of Consumer Studies, 34*, 587–595.

Butler, T., Richters, J., Yap, L., & Donovan, B. (2013). Condoms for prisoners: No evidence that they increase sex in prison, but they increase safe sex. *Sexually Transmitted Infections*. doi: 10.1136/sextrans-2012-050856

Caraher, M., Dixon, P., Carr-Hill, R., Hayton, P., McGough, H., & Bird, L. (2002). Are health-promoting prisons an impossibility? Lessons from England and Wales. *Health Education, 102*, 219–229.

Collica, K. (2002). Levels of knowledge and risk perceptions about HIV/AIDS among female inmates in New York state: Can prison-based HIV programs set the stage for behavior change? *The Prison Journal, 82*, 101–124.

Department of Health. (2002). *Health promoting prisons: A shared approach*. London: Crown.

Department of Health. (2009). *Improving health, supporting justice: The national delivery plan of the health and criminal justice programme board*. London: Author.

de Viggiani, N. (2006). A new approach to prison public health? Challenging and advancing the agenda for prison health. *Critical Public Health, 16*, 307–316.

de Viggiani, N. (2007). Unhealthy prisons: Exploring structural determinants of prison health. *Sociology of Health & Illness, 29*, 115–135.

de Viggiani, N., Orme, J., Powell, J., & Salmon, D. (2005). New arrangements for prison health care. *British Medical Journal, 330*, 918.

Dixey, R., Cross, R., Foster, S., & Woodall, J. (2013). Foundations of health promotion. In R. Dixey (Ed.), *Health promotion: Global principles and practice*. London: CABI.

Dooris, M. (2007). *Healthy settings: Past, present and future* (Unpublished PhD thesis). Deakin University, Victoria.

Dooris, M. (2009). Holistic and sustainable health improvement: The contribution of the settings-based approach to health promotion. *Perspectives in Public Health, 129*, 29–36.

Edgar, K., O'Donnell, I., & Martin, C. (2003). *Prison violence. The dynamics of conflict, fear and power*. Cullompton: Willan.

Edgar, K., Jacobson, J., & Biggar, K. (2011). *Time well spent: A practical guide to active citizenship and volunteering in prison*. London: Prison Reform Trust.

Fazel, S., & Danesh, J. (2002). Serious mental disorder in 23,000 prisoners: A systematic review of 62 surveys. *The Lancet, 359*, 545–550.

Freudenberg, N. (2001). Jails, prisons, and the health of urban populations: A review of the impact of the correctional system on community health. *Journal of Urban Health: Bulletin of the New York Academy of Medicine, 78*, 214–235.

Gatherer, A., Moller, L., & Hayton, P. (2005). The World Health Organization European health in prisons project after 10 years: Persistent barriers and achievements. *American Journal of Public Health, 95*, 1696–1700.

Gear, S. (2007). Behind the bars of masculinity: Male rape and homophobia in and about south african men's prisons. *Sexualities, 10*, 209–227.

Goffman, E. (1968). *Asylums: Essays on the social situation of mental patients*. Harmondsworth: Penguin.

Grinstead, O., Zack, B., Faigeles, B., Grossman, N., & Blea, L. (1999). Reducing postrelease HIV risk among male prison inmates: A peer-led intervention. *Criminal Justice and Behavior, 26*, 453–465.

Hayton, P. (2007). Protecting and promoting health in prisons: A settings approach. In L. Møller, H. Stöver, R. Jürgens, A. Gatherer, & H. Nikogosian (Eds.), *Health in prisons* (pp. 15–20). Copenhagen: WHO.

Hensley, C. (2000). Attitudes toward homosexuality in a male and female prison: An exploratory study. *The Prison Journal, 80*, 434–441.

Herbert, K., Plugge, E., Foster, C., & Doll, H. (2012). Prevalence of risk factors for non-communicable diseases in prison populations worldwide: A systematic review. *The Lancet, 379*, 1975–1982.

HM Prison Service. (2003). *Prison service order (PSO) 3200 on health promotion*. London: Author.

HMIP. (1996). *Patient or prisoner? A new strategy for health care in prisons*. London: Home Office.

Ireland, J. L. (2002). *Bullying among prisoners: Evidence, research and intervention strategies*. London: Routledge.

Ireland, C. A., & Ireland, J. L. (2000). Descriptive analysis of the nature and extent of bullying behavior in a maximum-security prison. *Aggressive Behavior, 26*, 213–223.

Jacobs, J. (1977). *Stateville*. Chicago, IL: University of Chicago Press.

Jarvis, J., Graham, S., Hamilton, P., & Tyler, D. (2004). The role of parenting classes for young fathers in prison: A case study. *Probation Journal, 51*, 21–33.

Kemm, J. (2001). Health impact assessment: A tool for healthy public policy. *Health Promotion International, 16*, 79–85.

Kickbusch, I. (1986). Issues in health promotion: Dr Ilona Kickbusch. *Health Promotion International, 1*, 437–442.

Kickbusch, I. (2003). The contribution of the World Health Organization to a new public health and health promotion. *American Journal of Public Health, 93*, 383–388.

Knepper, P. (2007). *Criminology and social policy*. London: Sage.

Lahm, K. F. (2009). Inmate assaults on prison staff: A multilevel examination of an overlooked form of prison violence. *The Prison Journal, 89*, 131–150.

Lehma, C. (2001). Description and evaluation of a health education program for women offenders. *The ABNF Journal, 12*, 124–129.

Lester, C., Hamilton-Kirkwood, L., & Jones, N. K. (2003). Health indicators in a prison population: Asking prisoners. *Health Education Journal, 62*, 341–349.

Levenson, J., & Farrant, F. (2002). Unlocking potential: Active citizenship and volunteering by prisoners. *Probation Journal, 49*, 195–204.

Levy, M. (2005). Prisoner health care provision: Reflections from Australia. *International Journal of Prisoner Health, 1*, 65–73.

Lincoln, T., Miles, J. R., & Scheibel, S. (2007). Community health and public health collaborations. In R. B. Greifinger, J. Bick, & J. Goldenson (Eds.), *Public health behind bars* (pp. 508–534). New York, NY: Springer.

Lines, R. (2006). From equivalence of standards to equivalence of objectives: The entitlement of prisoners to health care standards higher than those outside prisons. *International Journal of Prisoner Health, 2*, 269–280.

Link, B. G., & Phelan, J. C. (2002). McKeown and the idea that social conditions are fundamental causes of disease. *American Journal of Public Health, 92*, 730–732.

Magura, S., Kang, S. Y., & Shapiro, J. L. (1994). Outcomes of intensive AIDS education for male adolescent drug users in jail. *Journal of Adolescent Health, 15*, 457–463.

Marmot, M., Friel, S., Bell, R., Houweling, T. A., & Taylor, S. (2008). Closing the gap in a generation: Health equity through action on the social determinants of health. *The Lancet, 372*, 1661–1669.

Marquart, J. W., Merianos, D. E., Hebert, J. L., & Carroll, L. (1997). Health condition and prisoners: A review of research and emerging areas of inquiry. *The Prison Journal, 77*, 184–208.

Milio, N. (1986). *Promoting health through public policy*. Ottawa: Canadian Public Health Association.

Moller, L., Gatherer, A., & Dara, M. (2009). Barriers to implementation of effective tuberculosis control in prisons. *Public Health, 123*, 419–421.

Møller, L., Stöver, H., Jürgens, R., Gatherer, A., & Nikogosian, H. (2007). *Health in prisons*. Copenhagen: WHO.

Morris, T., & Morris, P. (1963). *Pentonville: A sociological study of an English prison*. London: Routledge.

Newton, C. (1994). Gender theory and prison sociology: Using theories of masculinities to interpret the sociology of prisons for men. *The Howard Journal of Criminal Justice, 33*, 193–202.

Niveau, G. (2007). Relevance and limits of the principle of "equivalence of care" in prison medicine. *Journal of Medical Ethics, 33*, 610–613.

Nutbeam, D. (1998). Evaluating health promotion – Progress, problems and solutions. *Health Promotion International, 13*, 27–44.

Nutbeam, D. (2008). What would the Ottawa charter look like if it were written today? *Critical Public Health, 18*, 435–441.

Phelan, J. C., Link, B. G., & Tehranifar, P. (2010). Social conditions as fundamental causes of health inequalities: Theory, evidence, and policy implications. *Journal of Health and Social Behavior, 51*(1 Suppl), S28–S40.

Plugge, E., Douglas, N., & Fitzpatrick, R. (2006). *The health of women in prison*. Oxford: Department of Public Health, University of Oxford.

Prison Reform Trust. (2009). *Bromley briefings. Prison fact file*. London: Author.

Ramaswamy, M., & Freudenberg, N. (2007). Health promotion in jails and prisons: An alternative paradigm for correctional health services. In R. B. Greifinger, J. Bick, & J. Goldenson (Eds.), *Public health behind bars* (pp. 229–248). New York, NY: Springer.

Reyes, H. (2001). Health and human rights in prison. In P. Bollini (Ed.), *HIV in prisons* (Ch. 2, pp. 9–18). Copenhagen: WHO.

Robertson, S. (2006). 'Not living life in too much of an excess': Lay men understanding health and well-being. *Health, 10*, 175–189.

Ross, M. (2013). *Health and health promotion in prisons*. Oxon: Routledge.

Ross, M., Harzke, A. J., Scott, D. P., McCann, K., & Kelley, M. (2006). Outcomes of project wall talk: An HIV/AIDS peer education program implemented within the Texas state prison system. *AIDS Education and Prevention, 18*, 504–517.

Rutherford, M., & Duggan, S. (2009). Meeting complex health needs in prisons. *Public Health, 123*, 415–418.

Rütten, A., & Gelius, P. (2011). The interplay of structure and agency in health promotion: Integrating a concept of structural change and the policy dimension into a multi-level model and applying it to health promotion principles and practice. *Social Science & Medicine, 73*, 953–959.

Salmon, S. (2005). Prisoners' children matter. *Prison Service Journal, 159*, 16–19.

Scott, D. P., Harzke, A. J., Mizwa, M. B., Pugh, M., & Ross, M. W. (2004). Evaluation of an HIV peer education program in Texas prisons. *Journal of Correctional Health Care, 10*, 151–173.

Senior, J., & Shaw, J. (2007). Prison healthcare. In Y. Jewkes (Ed.), *Handbook on prisons* (pp. 377–398). Cullompton: Willan.

Servan, A. K. (2012). *Societal reintegration experiences of women with judicial sentences participating in a re-entry program in Norway-from wrongdoings to wellbeing* (MSc thesis). Bergen: University of Bergen.

Shalev, S. (2008). *A sourcebook on solitary confinement*. London: Mannheim Centre for Criminology.

Sifunda, S., Reddy, P. S., Braithwaite, R., Stephens, T., Bhengu, S., Ruiter, R. A., & van den Borne, B. (2008). The effectiveness of a peer-led HIV/AIDS and STI health education intervention for prison inmates in South Africa. *Health Education & Behavior, 35*, 494–508.

Sim, J. (1990). *Medical power in prisons*. Milton Keynes: Open University Press.

Sim, J. (2002). The future of prison health care: A critical analysis. *Critical Social Policy, 22*, 300–323.

Smith, C. (2000). 'Healthy Prisons': A contradiction in terms? *The Howard Journal of Criminal Justice, 39*, 339–353.

Smith, C. (2002). Punishment and pleasure: Women, food and the imprisoned body. *Sociological Review, 50*, 197–211.

Social Exclusion Unit. (2002). *Reducing re-offending by ex-prisoners*. London: Crown.

Solomon, E. (2004). Criminals or citizens? Prisoner councils and rehabilitation. *Criminal Justice Matters, 56*, 24–25.

Solomon, E., & Edgar, K. (2004). *Having their say: The work of prisoner councils*. London: Prison Reform Trust.

South, J., Bagnall, A., Hulme, C., Woodall, J., Longo, R., Dixey, R., … Wright, J. (forthcoming). *A systematic review of the effectiveness and cost-effectiveness of peer-based interventions to maintain and improve offender health in prison settings* (Report for the National Institute for Health Research (NIHR) Health Services and Delivery Research (NIHR HS&DR) programme Project: 10/2002/13).

Spalek, B. (2002). *Islam, crime and criminal justice*. Cullompton: Willan.

Sparks, M. (2011). Building healthy public policy: Don't believe the misdirection. *Health Promotion International, 26*, 259–262.

Spencer, J., Haslewood-Pocsik, I., & Smith, E. (2009). 'Trying to get it right': What prison staff say about implementing race relations policy. *Criminology and Criminal Justice, 9*, 187–206.

Squires, N. (1996). Promoting health in prisons. *British Medical Journal, 313*, 1161.

Squires, P., & Measor, L. (2001). 'Breaking in': Partnership working, health promotion and prison walls. In D. Taylor (Ed.), *Breaking down barriers. Reviewing partnership practice* (pp. 124–164). Brighton: University of Brighton.

St Leger, L. (1997). Editorial. Health promoting settings: Form Ottawa to Jakarta. *Health Promotion International, 12*, 99–101.

Stewart, D. (2008). *The problems and needs of newly sentenced prisoners: Results from a national survey*. London: Ministry of Justice.

Svensson, S. (1996). Imprisonment – A matter of letting people live or stay alive? Some reasoning from a Swedish point of view. *Journal of Correctional Education, 47*, 69–72.

Sykes, G. M. (1958). *The society of captives: A study of a maximum security prison*. Princeton, NJ: Princeton University Press.

The Aldridge Foundation, & Johnson, M. (2008). *The user voice of the criminal justice system*. London: The Aldridge Foundation.

The Centre for Social Justice. (2009). *Breakthrough Britain: Locked up potential*. London: Author.

Visher, C. A., & Travis, J. (2003). Transitions from prison to community: Understanding individual pathways. *Annual Review of Sociology, 29*, 89–113.

Warwick-Booth, L., Cross, R., & Lowcock, D. (2012). *Contemporary health studies: An introduction*. Cambridge: Polity Press.

White, A., & Johnson, M. (2000). Men making sense of their chest pain – Niggles, doubts and denials. *Journal of Clinical Nursing, 9*, 534–541.

Whitehead, D. (2006). The health promoting prison (HPP) and its imperative for nursing. *International Journal of Nursing Studies, 43*, 123–131.

WHO. (1986). Ottawa charter for health promotion. *Health Promotion, 1*, iii–v. doi:10.1093/heapro/1.4.405

WHO. (1998). *Mental health promotion in prisons* (Report on a WHO meeting). Copenhagen: Author.

WHO. (2001a). *HIV in prisons. A reader with particular relevance to the newly independent states.* Geneva: Author.

WHO. (2001b). *Prisons, drugs and society. A consensus statement on principles, policies and practices.* Geneva: Author.

WHO. (2003). *Promoting the health of young people in custody.* Copenhagen: Author.

WHO. (2005). *Status paper on prisons, drugs and harm reduction.* Geneva: Author.

WHO. (2007). *Health in prisons. A WHO guide to the essentials in prison health.* Copenhagen: Author.

WHO. (2008). *Background paper for Trenčín statement on prisons and mental health.* Copenhagen: Author.

Winterbauer, N. L., & Diduk, R. M. (2013). The ten essential public health services model as a framework for correctional health care. *Journal of Correctional Health Care, 19*, 43–53.

Woodall, J. (2010a). *Control and choice in three category-C English prisons: Implications for the concept and practice of the health promoting prison* (Unpublished PhD thesis). Leeds Metropolitan University, Leeds.

Woodall, J. (2010b). Exploring concepts of health with male prisoners in three category-C English prisons. *International Journal of Health Promotion and Education, 48*, 115–122.

Woodall, J. (2012). Social and environmental factors influencing in-prison drug use. *Health Education, 112*, 31–46.

Woodall, J., & South, J. (2012). Health promoting prisons: Dilemmas and challenges. In A. Scriven & M. Hodgins (Eds.), *Health promotion settings: Principles and practice* (pp. 170–186). London: Sage.

Woodall, J., Dixey, R., Green, J., & Newell, C. (2009). Healthier prisons: The role of a prison visitors' centre. *International Journal of Health Promotion and Education, 47*, 12–18.

Woodall, J., Dixey, R., & South, J. (2013). Control and choice in English prisons: Developing health-promoting prisons. *Health Promotion International.* doi:10.1093/heapro/dat1019

Zack, B., Smith, C., Andrews, M. C., & May, J. P. (2013). Peer health education in Haiti's national penitentiary: The 'health through walls' experience. *Journal of Correctional Health Care, 19*, 65–68.

Index